THE
SKIN REGIME

BOOT CAMP
FOR BEAUTIFUL SKIN

DANA RAMOS
FOREWORD BY DR. DAVID BANK

ISBN: 0615653170
ISBN-13: 9780615653174

Library of Congress Control Number: 2012941466
Verve Productions, LLC, Goldens Bridge, NY

Published in the United States by Verve Productions
Printed by CreateSpace, an Amazon.com company

www.TheSkinRegime.com

CONTENTS:

iv

Eyes and eyebrows
Treating dark circles under the eyes
Treating red, irritated eyes
Lips
Bright teeth and sweet breath

Plastic surgery, lasers, lifts
Injectables: Botox, fillers
Oral Meds: Isotretinoin, Antibiotics
Unwanted hair removal
The truth about cellulite
Liposuction

Hair
Arms, Legs
Bumps on the back of arms and thighs, rough patches
  on knees and elbows
Hands, feet and nails
Perfumes
The neglected areas

Handy Take-With-You Shopping List

A CHALLENGE
TO MAJOR COSMETIC COMPANIES

"Oh, no you didn't"...

We at The Skin Regime would like to challenge any major drugstore or department store cosmetic/skin care line to go up against the glycolic products and techniques suggested in *The Skin Regime; Boot Camp for Beautiful Skin*.

We suggest taking a handful of women (and a man or two), have them use the Expensive Skin Care company's products on one side of their face, and The Skin Regime plan and ingredients/products mentioned on the other.

Then, after a few weeks, let us compare. If any company's products _even come close_ to the great results that can be accomplished <u>at home</u> with The Skin Regime, we will donate to their charities and promote them on our web and in future revisions.

If they fail, we get "bragging rights" and the company will donate to The Skin Cancer Foundation and other wonderful charities of our choice.

We bet none will take the challenge. Wanna know why? Read on!

Oh, yes we did! It's ON. Bring it!

Foreword by Dr. David Bank

I'm very pleased that my friend and patient, Dana Ramos, has written *The Skin Regime: Boot Camp for Beautiful Skin*. As a dermatologist, I am alarmed by the harm I witness in my office, such as people who don't protect their skin from the sun and arrive with severe damage or cancerous conditions, and the newest trend of people buying strong acid products off the internet and burning themselves because they aren't fully educated on how to safely use those products.

And I groan when I see people spend hundreds or thousands of dollars on bogus "miracle" creams that do nothing but waste your money.

I have made it a personal goal to inform people about harmful skincare practices and fraudulent products—and to show them how great skin can absolutely be accomplished using inexpensive products, or medically-accepted and proven methods—methods that are used widely by reputable physicians, and really work.

In this book, Dana Ramos uses humor and in-your-face bluntness to tell the truth about skincare—and sometimes that means telling you what can NOT be attained (at least, not yet) either by products or medical intervention—for instance, *The Skin Regime* reveals the truth about cellulite treatments.

More truth—you can get great skin with inexpensive methods, right in your own home.

Another truth—sometimes people have skin issues that cannot be battled at home—like cystic acne or severe rosacea. But thankfully, those disfiguring conditions can also be treated medically, painlessly, and often inexpensively by dermatologists armed with the latest inventions in skincare, like lasers that can remove or improve scars, wrinkles, and more.

The Skin Regime is a no-holds-barred guide to truth versus fiction. Stop wasting your money on useless products, and find out what you can really accomplish on your own, or with the help of a physician.

Sincerely,

Dr. David Bank
June, 2012

PART ONE

Introduction to The Skin Regime

That is an UNTOUCHED-UP PHOTO of me, Dana, on the back cover of The Skin Regime and on the website: I have on no makeup base or foundation-just moisturizers. Really—that is *my* skin in full bright sunlight wearing only eye makeup and lip color. No blush, no cover-up, no retouching, no air-brushing-nothing. Not even taken by a pro photographer—just a good close-up and a little Sony camera that fits in your pocket.

At age 49.

People come up to me all the time—mostly people I have never met—and comment on my "gorgeous" skin and ask me what products I use. Or they say how lucky I am to have such great *genes* that gave me such great skin.

I'm flattered of course—but *lucky*? No, dear. I WAS NOT BORN WITH GREAT SKIN. Far from it. It took me years to learn how to battle numerous skin problems and discover what worked to cure them. And furthermore, I learned what would work *beyond* just curing my skin problems—I wanted to know how to attain truly great, dewy, glowing skin.

Those of us involved with *The Skin Regime* are committed to telling you the TRUTH about skin care and skin care products.

Here is the truth: You can have great skin at any age and you don't have to spend a lot of money.

Why did you write this book?

For you, for myself, and for good causes.

I came up with *The Skin Regime* concept because people were asking me how, at my age, I had such great and youthful-looking skin. I began spending a lot of time chatting to people at the gym or in stores, and writing long, explanatory emails or on phone calls telling friends—and some people I barely knew—about my skin story and how to get great skin. Sometimes I would simply say, "Just go see a good dermatologist." But a lot of people didn't want to spend the time and expense for a doctor if they could do something on their own.

They just wanted to know my personal regime.

Finally, a light bulb went off and I figured I might as well write down everything I learned over the years from my own doctors and let the average person make their own decisions on what they want to try, or not try.

After you read all the truth, you'll be armed and ready to decide whether you want to do-it-yourself to get great skin at home, or you'd prefer to attain great skin under the care of a good cosmetic dermatologist.

Kind of like deciding if you want to just take up jogging to get in physical shape, or work out with a trainer.

I also decided to write *The Skin Regime* for myself. I figured I might as well make a few dollars for the time and effort spent telling people about my skin care regime. Now, when someone asks, "Tell me all about how you got such great skin," I can just give them the book or tell them to go to the website.

It bothers me to see people getting ripped off with phony creams and promises made by some companies. I want to get the truth out there.

And all of us at *The Skin Regime* are committed to help make the world a better place by reaching out to good causes and worthwhile non-profits and donating some of our proceeds toward them.

What is *The Skin Regime*?

THE SKIN REGIME: Boot Camp for Beautiful Skin reveals simple truths and formulas that will get your skin into shape in just weeks—the way a fitness regime would get your body in shape if you worked out for several weeks.

Think of it as "boot camp for the skin."

After you get your great skin, I explain how you can easily maintain it.

Do you have "bad," "not so great," or "blah" skin? Maybe some breakouts, or discoloration due to age or sun-damage or hormone changes? Fine lines, old acne scars, spots, uneven tone, large pores? Dull or dry skin?

Did you ever wish you could just scrape away the top layers and get glowing, natural, healthy skin?

So did I.

You've tried so many creams and preparations and promises. You're embarrassed that you fell for the charming and enthusiastic sales pitch in the department store and bought the Expensive Skin Care Line that ultimately disappointed you.

And you have done that more than once, right? You have wished you could get back the money on all the preparations you have tried over the years. I bet you'd have enough to buy a new car with all that wasted money.

You *wanted* to believe in the medical-sounding products you saw heavily advertised in magazines or on TV. The "Doctor-this" or "Doctor-that" Skin Care Line, The "New" or "Revolutionary," or "Secret" formulas showing fake or touched-up photos on infomercials with heavily-made-up actresses swearing this was the "greatest," the "best."

You wanted your latest purchases to really work, for once. You were seduced, you fell for it. You thought if it said "doctor recommended" or "clinically proven" or "all-natural," it would work—it would really *really* work. This one would be the *one.*

But you ended up frustrated and disappointed—again.

Yeah, so did I.

4

There are hundreds of competing products and skincare lines out there. And most of them so *expensive,* some ridiculously over-priced! There is a vast array of dermatology and skincare websites and books and articles in magazines—and they all have different products they are pushing.

You wish you knew what really works, and wished it didn't cost so much. But you've given up on all the promises. You don't even want to put out the effort anymore.

Yeah, that's how I felt, too.

Well, here's the thing. For the most part, those good-looking, seductive lounge-lizards products simply entice you and betray you—but there *really are* products that work. And they are reasonably priced if you know what it is you are looking for and where to get them.

And this is the bottom-line truth: *It is all about the key ingredients in the products, not the name on the product.* Even though the Expensive Skin Care Lines *sometimes* contain those key ingredients, they are most likely just low-strength preparations dropped in luscious-looking glass jars. You end up paying for a watered-down impotent product—and very little of it—in pretty packaging that cost more than the key ingredients.

The reason these companies don't make their products with *effective* strength is because they are going after as many consumers as possible and they don't want to deal with complaints and product returns from mild side-effects that are NORMAL when you begin using the products (such as some irritation, or a possible temporary increase in breakouts). The companies just want the largest bottom-line consumer base to make the most money possible.

Those products with low-strength key ingredients will not do the job, and many other "special ingredients" are just bogus or unproven substances that do virtually nothing for your skin. Usually, it is all about some passing fad, like some fruit or berry or other food-item allegedly "discovered" for skin benefits, or caffeine, or chocolate, or mud.

And collagens—that are used in all those anti-aging preparations? Ask any honest doctor: You can't implant collagen in skin with a cream any more than you can remove cellulite in a cream (more on that in Part Five of this book).

There are some absurd products that uses crushed or liquefied gold in skin preparations. And what exactly does anyone expect from wasting money like that? According to most dermatologists, you are more likely to end up with irritated skin at worst, and nothing at best.

The list of lies, fakes, phonies and frauds are so long, it would take another book just to write about them.

But this is not a book about all the baloney and bogus stuff out there, this is a book about THE TRUTH and WHAT NEARLY EVERY DERMATOLOGIST AGREES are the ingredients and methods that absolutely ARE effective, that can help you get great skin, healthy skin, glowing skin.

Getting great skin is about knowing how to use the right ingredients in the proper combination for results. You need a regime (some people call it a *regimen*)—just like you would need a diet or exercise routine to shape up your body.

The Skin Regime: Boot Camp for Beautiful Skin, takes only a few minutes a week—and only for a few weeks of diligence—to develop an entire new look and feel for your skin.

The Skin Regime uses guerrilla tactics, too: Attacking your skin problems quickly and effectively with a few critical products that really get in and get the job done. It reveals the important working active ingredients—they are generic ingredients—and how to use them. This way, you can find your own favorites in preparations with the proper strength.

We have also created a website where you can find information and resources on these inexpensive products: TheSkinRegime.com. Feel free to explore product brands you feel best suits you. For the Peels, we encourage you to call the respectable companies and ask for sample sizes and information on how to use their particular products. Tell them you heard about them from The Skin Regime—a widely-read website—and that you hope to report favorably about them to us. Hey, in this day and age, you deserve to have the best customer-service experience and we want to know if there is a company out there who should—or should not—be on our list of "recommendations."

Once you learn read about the essential ingredients and products that really work and start acquiring your favorites, just be sure you deal with trusted companies who have been selling their products at least for a few years. And we know you've been burned so many times—so we encourage you to get on the web and compare other reputable companies and prices to assure yourself.

Remember: There is no such thing as a "secret" ingredients that really work. The effective products are no secret at all.

Remember, too, that all skin is individual. You must find products with the right strength for your skin-type, and do patch-tests of all preparations and products before you put them on your face.

I'll explain it all in this simple, direct, honest book.

I'm going to sweep away all the clutter and expense and tell you the *truth* about the products and the *truth* about what works and what to do to get amazing, glowing, baby-butt smooth skin—for far less money than you would have to spend with cosmetic treatments and facials at skin-care centers.

Wait a minute. Are you saying all facial treatments at doctor's offices or salons are bogus?

No. They are not all bogus, though *some* are. You'll understand the difference after reading *The Skin Regime*. If you use a trusted cosmetic dermatologist, you can be pretty sure he or she is using great products.

There will always be people who need or want to go to dermatologists, or those who simply prefer having a pro give them facials and peels. Just like some people prefer to have manicures at a salon, whereas some do their nails themselves (and more on that in Part Six of this book!)

Some people need much stronger treatments for more unusual skin issues that simply must be handled by a physician—and you may be one of them. After reading *The Skin Regime*, you'll be able to make that decision.

But many people simply don't have the kind of time and money to go to fancy doctors and salons. And worse—a lot of people are burning their skin by buying stuff on the internet and trying to do things themselves without knowing what they are really buying or how to do things properly. Then, they end up HAVING to go to a dermatologist to fix the damage!

We're committed to telling the truth about skincare, and that includes letting you know what you can do yourself, safely. You can then use the money you save on exploring other treatments you may want—such as for Botox or injectable fillers (more on that coming up, too!) Or new clothes!

If all the stuff out there is fake or useless, how can these companies make the claims and advertise like they do? Won't the government crack down on them?

Our government agencies can barely keep track of much more important issues in our country, and you think they have the resources to go after companies that make you believe you are going to get a facelift from a jar, or lose weight by taking a bogus capsule, or achieve "male enhancement" from a cream or pill? Sure, if some product starts killing people the regulators will get on the job, but they can't go after every fraudulent claim out there. Regulatory agencies like the Food and Drug Administration and the Federal Trade Commission simply can't keep up with the outrageous claims and false advertising that skin-care products make any more than they can stop those other outrageous and hyper-promised products. And by the time they get around to slapping the wrist of a deceitful company, the hoaxer wriggles out with a slight change of name or advertising, or they modify their claims a little.

For instance, a hoax ad might claim, "According to medical experts, this cream will lift and rejuvenate your skin." Which it won't, but if they even get caught, maybe they get a slap on the wrist. So they promise not to advertise that again. A new slogan will then say, "According to medical experts, this cream may lift and rejuvenate your skin."

Did you catch the difference? One little word-switch of "will" to "may."

There are numerous examples of that sort of hoaxing word-play in skin care, diet products, hair restoration products, male enhancement ads, etc. And even in politics!

Too many businesses thrive on this sort of nonsense, but if you believe that a cream will give you results like a surgical face-lift, or remove cellulite, then it is time for a reality check.

I understand the desire to believe—we all want to believe in miracles, or that a product will do what it promises to do. But stop wasting money on delusions and fantasies. You'll feel better when you get results from the indisputable products that actually *do* work and live up to the claims.

You don't have to believe us—just get on the web, or visit a trusted and certified dermatologist and ask about various ingredients and products. In the appendix of this book, I list some resources if you want to get the really techno medical sources and geek info on this stuff. There is simply no denying the evidence and truth.

And you probably don't want to hear this either, but you know those "all natural," "preservative-free," "holistic," and other whatever-is-the-latest-buzz-word products that come out with claims and so-called "clinical trials?" Much all of it is bull. Bull, bull and more bull. First of all, many *chemicals* can be called "all natural," because they are essentially derived from nature. And many self-proclaimed all-natural products are actually harmful! You also need to consider that some common herbal products and vitamins can have far more harmful effects than the chemicals used for skin care. When used properly, chemical preparations can be safer than what you find in a health-food store.

And lest we forget—plenty of people have allergies to all-natural products (peanuts, pollen, etc.), and nobody likes the all-natural plant called Poison Ivy. If you think "all natural" or "holistic" automatically translates to meaning "better," you are gravely mistaken.

Get honest with yourself: You use hair products, deodorants, nail polish, tons of body lotions. You drink wine, breathe modern-day air, eat processed foods and vegetables grown with chemical intervention—no matter how much you try, you can't get away from all this. You drink sodas and caffeinated beverages, eat candy and brush your teeth with a toothpaste filled with ingredients that sound like they should be used in nuclear reactors instead of something you put in your mouth. But you want to worry about a little bit of a product containing a little bit of a chemical that you put on your *face?* You probably poison yourself a hundred times worse by eating a bag of Cheezy Chips than you would with months worth of the facial products listed in this book.

Have you taken an honest look at *your* face?

Have you really looked at your face the way other people see you during the day? In other words—not just in front of a bathroom mirror? Grab a mirror and walk over to a bright window. Better yet, step outdoors.

Take a good look.

Yes, that is what your skin really looks like. The makeup really shows *that* much, the skin really is *that* uneven.

Now take a look at a part of your skin that has never seen the sun—like your breasts or your butt. Surely there has to be *someplace* on your body that has never seen the light of day? (Maybe you better go back inside before you do this check).

You see how smooth and nice the un-sun-touched skin is? Do you realize that *all the skin on your body* would look like those hidden places if your skin had been cared for properly and protected your entire life?

Don't cry over the past: Following *The Skin Regime* can repair a lot of the damage you have done to your face, and get back much more gorgeous skin. But you will have to follow the plan, which means no more sitting out baking yourself in the sun.

More on that in a bit.

How long does *The Skin Regime* take?

With a time investment of only a few minutes or seconds each day, you will notice a positive difference in the first two weeks, and a *major* difference in six to twelve weeks. When you have attained the great skin you want, you will go on Maintenance and your skin will continue to improve with proper care. Maintenance will take only seconds a day.

What about the food I eat? Do I have to give up chocolate and fried foods or go on a special diet?

No. This is not a diet book. Furthermore, the "some foods cause acne" myth has been largely debunked, as the medical geek sites and any modern dermatologist will confirm. Chocolate and fried foods really don't make acne worse for most people. We encourage a healthy diet of good foods and vitamins for overall health and beauty, but you do NOT have to do any special diet for *The Skin Regime* to gain remarkable benefits for your skin.

Try to drink a good amount of water each day for proper hydration and many other health benefits.

Is it all about the face?

No, we don't stop at the face! The skin organ covers your entire body, and there are trouble spots everywhere, so we address the entire body. We focus on the face first and foremost because that is what 99 percent of people see first.

Your face is your calling-card, the first thing people see and evaluate about you, and most important for first impressions. And your face is the reason you picked up this book—having dewy elbows is not the most important thing to you.

But be assured, *The Skin Regime* will also reveal how to get great smooth lips, elbows, hands, and feet. We'll tell you how to get rid of those pimply bumps on the back of your arms and butt and thighs and how to get an all-over smooth, glowing body that feels better, looks better, and feels nice to touch.

And there will be some facts and tips about getting smooth shine to your hair.

All with products that cost a fraction of what it costs with those Expensive Skin Care products.

Who Can Use *The Skin Regime*?

Anyone at any age—who is NOT PREGNANT.

If you have moderately troubled skin <u>without</u> severe skin problems such as cystic acne or lesions or hypersensitivity—*The Skin Regime* will most likely improve your skin dramatically.

Is it hard to do *The Skin Regime*?

Look, we're no rocket scientists and we can do it ourselves, and have been for years.

If you can read and follow simple instructions then you can do it, too. The Peels described in *The Skin Regime* are mild and designed to work over several weeks, they are NOT heavy-duty chemical peels that should only be administered by a doctor. But with this gentle Peel regime spread over several weeks, you'll get similar or possibly better effects than those harsher one-time only treatments.

There is nothing brand-new in this book; *The Skin Regime* is based on many dermatological and medical/esthetic skin facials that use the same ingredients and often the exact same products. Having facial peels through a dermatologist or "medical" skin store or spa costs thousands of dollars because you need to do several facials over the course of several weeks. One is not enough. *And at $150-200 for each facial, plus home-care products?* Well that adds up to quite a bit of time and money.

With *The Skin Regime,* you can get great results with much of same common ingredients and the same science behind the methods.

Don't forget—we are talking about the popular mild facials and peels that dermatologists, estheticians and salons do—not the heavy-duty one-time peels that use caustic levels of chemicals and are designed to create a drastic peels that takes days or weeks to heal. Those types are often done by specially-trained physicians to treat severe issues and scar removal. Sometimes a plastic surgeon will do it along with a facelift.

Even though there are companies that sell strong acids that can burn your skin like that—you must never attempt such drastic measures at home. If you have severely scarred skin that needs a strong fix, you must seek improvement through licensed physicians trained in these procedures.

So: *The Skin Regime* will improve your skin tremendously, but is too mild to remove <u>severe</u> scars or wrinkles.

Research shows that no two dermatology experts agree on *every* single aspect about skin care, but virtually *all agree* that the main products listed in this book REALLY DO what they say they will and that these products have revolutionized skin care. They *all agree* about the severe damaging effects of the sun on skin. Disagreement is usually about the newer and less-tested products that show promise, but have not been overwhelmingly proven to work. *The Skin Regime* does not include "promising" products, only the absolutely-proven ones. But, like following a diet, you do so at your own risk, reward and liability.

The Skin Regime is not a facelift (no duh), and won't lift sagging skin (no cream on earth can do that, only surgery). *The Skin Regime* cannot fill out deep lines like injectable fillers can.

But *The Skin Regime* can improve the tone and look of your skin significantly, and many fine lines should disappear. The typical follower of *The Skin Regime* will diminish discoloration, dullness, large pores, age spots and sunspots. Noticeably. Very noticeably, not the *"honey, I'm not sure… do you see a difference?"* kind of improvement. Check out some of the un-retouched photos on the TheSkinRegime.com for examples.

If you are already going to salons or skin spas and it *isn't* working for you, then try *The Skin Regime*—the products your facialist is using may *not* be the ones that really work. Read this book, then ask them what they are using so you can compare and make decisions going forward.

What if my skin is pretty good, I just want to keep it that way, or make it a little better?

We have plenty of suggestions that don't involve doing Peels—or maybe doing a mild Peel once in a while. If you read *The Skin Regime*, at least you'll know if you are wasting money on products you don't need or on expensive products that can be replaced with better, less-expensive ones. And—you'll learn what you might be doing that is really bad for your skin, and how to prevent problems in the future!

What about guys?

Guys are really getting into looking better these days, aren't they? In 18th century Europe and America, they used lots of makeup and wore powdered wigs and frilly clothing that were incredibly fussy and silly, and then they seemed to go back to cavemen days—where they stayed a long long time. A very long time. Very.

Thank heaven that's changing again. Guys often hate to admit they are taking special steps to look and feel better about their appearance. And they don't want to use "women's stuff"—so cosmetic companies slap a man-label on their moisturizers and the guys think they are getting something different or made in some sort of manly way for manly skin. Sometimes there are higher concentrations of some ingredients of some products, but mostly—it's psychology. Kind of like how guys call their handbags "messenger bags," because there is *no way* they are ever gonna admit they are carrying a purse!

It's okay guys—you can buy this book. You can follow *The Skin Regime* and get better skin. But a problem could come up with your shaving ritual. While you're in the "boot camp" phase of Peels, you might like to switch to an electric razor in order to avoid irritating your skin—those multiple-blade razors they make these days can cut real close and irritate your skin.

If you do follow *The Skin Regime*, use only moisturizing lotion as your lather and after-shave. Once your skin has been through the Peels phase and you are on Maintenance, you can return to your regular razors, although it is best to get rid of any alcohol-based after-shave.

 Warning: *The Skin Regime* is NOT for people with severe or cystic acne, open lesions on the skin, or issues of hyper-sensitivity to skin products. If you have rosacea (chronic red and bumpy patches on the skin), psoriasis, eczema, or another illness, you should first see a dermatologist to correct your severe issues. Afterwards, you can begin *The Skin Regime* to take your skin to the next level of greatness.

No Sunbathing! If you are hooked on sun tanning or tanning salons—put this book down *immediately* and come back when you come to your senses! You ended up with problems thanks mostly to sun damage, and *The Skin Regime* will help reverse the effects of that damage and give you a fresh start. However, it will leave your skin vulnerable for *even worse* damage by the sun if you expose your new, lovely skin to harmful, skin-ruining rays. Would you put a baby in the sun without sun protection? Of course not! So you must not do that to your skin, ever again. Be committed to using sunscreen if you will be in the sun more than a couple of minutes. If you cannot make this commitment, please do not use the products and techniques in this book.

If you are pregnant or thinking of becoming pregnant: Please wait until after you have the baby before using the products or beginning *The Skin Regime.* Some of the products are safe for pregnancy, some are *maybe* safe, and some are not. But why take the chance? And you may develop hormonal discoloration and other issues during or after the pregnancy. *The Skin Regime* will be there to fix your skin afterwards, so put this book on the shelf with the books that tell you how to change a diaper or find time for sex-after-baby. Can't hurt to wait until you are finished breast-feeding, too. We'll wait for you.

Do I have to use only the products you list for *The Skin Regime* to work?

If you want to spend money on luxury moisturizers and makeup because it makes you feel good—well it depends. After all, a massage won't cure you of tension forever, but it makes you feel good and it is harmless and has positive benefits. You may have some body lotions you just love and want to keep using. It's your money; knock yourself out. But to get great skin, make sure you go for the *key ingredients and strength of preparations* of the products listed in *The Skin Regime*. And we strongly suggest avoiding anything with perfumes or extraneous ingredients because it can really irritate your new "baby" skin. Stick with the products suggested in this book and you'll be playing it safe.

Can I wear my makeup while doing *The Skin Regime*?

Absolutely. You may wish to make adjustments to different kinds of makeup as your skin begins to change. And after your skin is glowing, you will probably want to show it off by going "nude." We'll discuss makeup and give some nononsense recommendations in this book.

Is *The Skin Regime* Safe?

We think what you want to ask is, "Is this safe to do *at home?*" The answer is, "Yes, if you use common sense and follow directions carefully." Follow the instructions carefully, don't overdo it, and use common sense—just as if you were taking a new vitamin or medicine or starting a diet. You will know when you need to back off something that might be over-irritating your skin or if it is not working as it should. We'll also remind you to test all products on parts of your body before trying on your face, as a precaution. We'll suggest modifications for people with different skin types.

Of course, even in a dermatologist or skincare office, there are no guarantees that you won't have an allergic or bad reaction. Everyone is different—whether you are trying a new diet or exercise regime, you never know until you start if you will be that one in a hundred that needs a modification from what works for the other 99 people. That is why you must use your common sense.

What about the science behind *The Skin Regime*?

This is not a textbook on skin care! You can get plenty of geek and techno info on a lot of websites, and there are some great books written by doctors which go into all the medical terms like *dermis*, *epidermis* and *subcutaneous* (your eyes are already glazing, right?). Those sites and books go into all the reasons why the products do what they do. I list favorite resources in the appendix of this book if you want to explode your brain by reading the medical literature. The point of this book is to cut to the chase and give you basic cold, hard facts and info you need to get your skin looking terrific in a few weeks. This is boot camp, baby!

The Truth about Expensive Skin Products:

Boy, are some Expensive Skin Care companies are going to be upset with me for writing this book! But the truth about those expensive creams and cosmetics? You are paying for the advertising, the name, the marketing, and the salaries of everyone working at the company.

Expensive brand-name products often contain some ingredients that work, but not in the essential percentages that work. And using more of a product will not "add up" to the correct percentage. A 15 SPF sunscreen plus another 15 SPF sunscreen does NOT add up to 30, even if you put on two layers—or more!

Example of a revelation that will tick them off: There is virtually no difference between well-made glycolic-acid preparations—expensive or inexpensive. But there is a big difference in strength (potency) depending on the percentage of glycolic acid used and the buffering agents used to make the preparations less reactive with the skin. The same is often true with well-prepared products that contain the other important ingredients that you need for *The Skin Regime*. Often, the same factories make the *exact same cosmetics* for dozens of companies—they just slap different brand names on the products. And they certainly slap on different prices, depending on how glitzy the brand-name is and how much they had to pay for the fancy jars and fancy marketing, not to mention the multi-million dollar contract for the celebrity spokesperson! We personally believe they also mark up the price if the name sounds French, but that is an undocumented theory.

And about those celebrities? Many of them are probably going for expensive skin treatments or to cosmetic dermatologists that perform very similar or identical techniques we reveal here in *The Skin Regime*. Those stars aren't getting that skin just from the products they promote. Very few people are born with genetically fantastic skin. We have to work at it, and so do they.

And don't forget—the ads of celebrities you see in the magazines are airbrushed beyond reality. There are even some lawsuits going on because of some misleading ads!

NONE OF THE PHOTOS OF THE SKIN that we feature in *The Skin Regime* and on our web are airbrushed or touched-up. NONE.

You can see what real skin looks like on real people—and what the Peels look like during the peeling phase, and after the "boot camp" phase when more glowing, radiant skin emerges.

Why don't most of the expensive and brand-name skin care products work as well as those described in *The Skin Regime*?

Simply because the brand-name products cannot make the products strong enough if they are going to market to a wide consumer base. If they did make them strong enough, they would have to write a whole book (like this one) explaining exactly how and why the products work and how to use them and what to expect. That would be a marketing night-mare for these companies that are going after mass-market consumers! They don't want to spend time dealing with people who have questions about why their skin is flaking or turning red during a peel, or explain how to make adjustments in products and how to maintain their skin. And without the explanations, people will use the products and return them, thinking something is "wrong." That would be unacceptable for these companies; they want to spend as little time as possible, reach as many consumers as possible, get as wide a base of sales as possible. Their approach: Just shut up and buy the stuff and you'll look like Halle Berry or Nicole Kidman.

We're not saying those products are all useless—some of them can work pretty well for Maintenance if you know what to look for. But why bother when you can get products that are far less expensive and work far better for you—products we will tell you about in *The Skin Regime.*

This book will tell you *exactly* what to look for in your preparations and how to find the best preparations for the least price. Sometimes, the best stuff at the best price comes right off the discount shelves of the drugstore or supermarket. We'll tell you everything you need to know.

A Word to Dermatologists and Other Skin Estheticians:

I know you are not happy that I'm revealing the low-priced in-home way for people to get great skin. I'm like a disloyal magician's assistant writing a tell-all book on how you do your magic tricks.

Because I'm giving away the blueprints to the magic tricks, some of you will denounce *The Skin Regime* and insist that people should "not try this at home." You will insist they must come to you instead. Don't be a hater! I love you guys and gals and I repeatedly suggest that anyone who has concerns and questions, anyone who is unsure of trying something on their own, anyone who has severe discoloration, severe acne, hyper-sensitivity or other troubling conditions, should *go to a dermatologist who specializes in cosmetic dermatology*. I give all the warnings and caveats as I go along, so relax. I'm not taking any business away from you—I'm writing this book for people who don't want to spend a fortune to get expensive treatments, or who don't have the time to deal with office visits.

If I have severe skin issues, why do you suggest a dermatologist and not an esthetician or facialist?

If you have severe skin problems or hypersensitivity, you really should see a dermatologist—a medical doctor who is highly trained to treat a variety of skin issues, including skin cancer. Facialists and estheticians are trained to give *facials*, not to treat severe issues. They can be helpful, but they are not trained to cure skin illness or disease. And many of them are worthless if they aren't using the products that are effective.

Dermatology as a medical specialty used to focus solely on skin diseases, rashes, and pimples. Now, with all the new ways to improve skin and reverse sun damage, many have expanded into everything from treating skin problems to injecting Botox and using lasers for purely cosmetic purposes. Not all dermatologists are *cosmetic dermatologists*, although the field is moving rapidly in that direction. When you call a potential dermatologist be sure to ask if they have all the new bells and whistles for cosmetic care and not only a practice that treats skin disease.

Dana's skin story:

I swear to you, I was not born with great skin. In fact, I suffered with bad skin and acne until I was 32 years old. Okay, yes—I was *born* with great skin like most babies are, but starting at age eleven, I began breaking out with pimples. Lots. And then breaking out more as each year progressed into adolescence. I tried everything: All the over-the-counter preparations, and whatever they had in the dermatological arsenal of the 1970's: Antibiotics, various acne creams, and bizarre treatments involving dry ice and sun lamps to name a few.

In my teens I was told, "You'll grow out of it." I slathered on thick makeup to try to hide the breakouts. But you know what that looks like—a girl with thick, caking makeup over bumpy skin. Lovely.

Then in my 20's I was told, "Its hormonal, you'll get past it." It was a constant struggle. Staying on antibiotics forever is a horrible idea, and didn't work all that well anyway, so I stopped taking them. And I still tried every new cream or gel that entered the medical arsenal—but to little effect.

In the 1980's a fabulous new cream came to the arsenal: Retin-A (known generically as *tretinoin*). It helped with acne, and also with some fine-lines and sun damage. But I still had breakouts and lots of uneven tone and large pores, etcetera. *Tretinoin* is a fantastic product (more on this later), but not enough weaponry for a complete acne cure or to get the great skin I hoped for.

By the time I hit my thirties, I was completely fed up with my skin and sick of wasting money from trying everything that offered hope. And I remember one day my husband asked, "What is that dirty stuff on your face?"

Dirty stuff?

"Yeah, it's like the sides of your face has smudgy dirt or something. Like light-brown skin sideburns, sort of."

When I got home I used two mirrors to get good side views of my face. What fresh hell was *this*? It certainly did look like dirty brown patches. Damn. And what would the future bring next—was I going to grow a *beard*? (Yes, I would actually. We'll talk about hair removal in Part Five in this book, dearies).

The "dirty spots" you might have or have seen on other people is known as *melasma*: Darker irregular patches of skin caused by hormonal changes or sun damage. I hadn't realized how bad the melasma spots had become because I didn't see myself in side-view, and my melasma was most prominent along the side of my face and jaw (common areas for it to appear), as well as one large spot on my forehead that I was always trying to cover with makeup.

I started doing some research again, and discovered some new products the medical community was enthusiastic about. But I faced a tough decision—I'd already gambled and lost so much money on products that didn't work very well and hated the thought of throwing out more money. And the disappointment, over and over!

But maybe the 1, 473rd time is the "charm."

> If you suffer severe acne or cystic acne, go to a good dermatologist and see what options you have for prescription medications. *Isotretinoin* is not for everyone, and still only available via prescription – and for good reason, such as it can cause birth defects in pregnant women. But used correctly, it is safe and effective.

I went to see a dermatologist in Los Angeles, and said, "Zits *and* wrinkles? Not fair! And these dirty-looking patches on my skin? Not acceptable." The doctor informed me that since I was not pregnant or planning any more babies in the near future, I might be a good candidate for a strong acne medication now generically known as *isotretinoin* (currently marketed under the brand names Accutane, Sotret, Claravis, and Amnesteem).

Isotretinoin is a powerful and miraculous oral medication for people who have bad acne, frequent breakouts and especially for that scourge called "cystic acne" that manifests with painful, deep and inflamed nodes under the skin. There is nothing the inflicted person can do about getting those cysts—they come from deep within the skin and it doesn't matter what you eat or drink or put on your face. These nodules can leave long-lasting scars and they cause a great deal of embarrassment and frustration.

I would get those kinds of nodules at least once a month, based on my hormonal cycles, but *isotretinoin* ended my breakouts—all of them. Whereas nothing else had ever truly worked for my acne, *isotretinoin* did. I was told that after a year or two, I might begin to get some breakouts again (I did) but that they would be easier to control (it was).

Okay, so after *isotretinoin*, I was in my thirties and had no zits, but was left with old acne scars, hormonal discoloration (those *dirty spots*), dull skin and brown spots. And some fine lines beginning to show on my face. Encouraged by my first success of getting my acne under control, I was eager to try some of the newer products, such as *alpha hydroxy* or *glycolic acid* peels, in order to improve the overall texture and appearance of my skin.

I continued my skin-care odyssey after I moved to the East Coast.

And so began my journey of learning what products are widely available, and what really works. I can say that my skin looks far better at age 51 than it did at age 32, or even 22. Sure, I have some well-earned lines—I am not trying to hide my age. Hiding age never works that well anyway—what works is improving your appearance so you look better and feel better about your appearance.

Facial lines give character—trying to erase all of them is unrealistic and simply looks bad—or even freaky if you go overboard. Knowing where to "draw the line" on *your* facial lines is a process of personal choice and learning what is available so you can make those choices. I'll discuss choices later—first you need to get your skin in great shape.

Okay, enough of my story. Let us get to work to make *your* great skin happen!

The Skin Regime is *not* about hiding your age, it is about having the best skin at any age. It is about minimizing acne, lines and discoloration because good skin looks *good*, not because it looks younger.

PART TWO

Creating Your New Skin
with The Skin Regime

 Let's preview some basic and critical points:

1. Do not become impatient. Skin needs time to regenerate between the Peels and rushing the process can cause damage or irritation that will slow down your progress.
2. Do not pick at your skin. This can also cause damage and irritation.
3. Keep the Peels separated by at least 7 – 14 days. We will explain how to know when to do each Peel, and when to stay on Maintenance.
4. No more sunbathing without complete ray-blocking sunscreen.
5. Do not practice *The Skin Regime* if you are pregnant or trying to get pregnant or if you have other medical issues that could be impacted.

6. Do not use if you have severe acne, hypersensitive skin, open skin lesions or other severe skin issues. *The Skin Regime* will help moderate acne tremendously, but it is not designed for severe issues that should be addressed with a dermatologist.

7. You may get so excited with the products that you'll think, "Why not use them all over my body?" Do NOT do this. These products are medical products and like any good medicine, you CAN overdose because the skin absorbs many medicines and chemicals to some degree. Follow *The Skin Regime* instructions and don't overdo it.

8. If anything unusual crops up or you have an adverse reaction, stop *The Skin Regime* and see a dermatologist to help you with your skin plan.

9. ALWAYS DO A PATCH TEST ON ANY PRODUCT BEFORE USING. Put a small amount behind an ear and another on inside of your arm near elbow and wait 24-48 hours to be sure your skin does not overreact or has an allergy to the product. THIS GOES FOR GLYCOLIC PREPARATIONS AS WELL AS ANY OVER-THE-COUNTER PREPARATIONS, including creams you buy in the drugstore.

 Important! This chapter focuses on safe, do-it-yourself "Peels," with glycolic acid preparation. This is a marvelous way to get terrific skin in a short time—

BUT IT IS NOT THE ONLY WAY. Read through this chapter, maybe even try a Peel or two. But if you decide you don't need or want Peels as part of your own Skin Regime, KEEP READING. Our chapter on Maintenance is for you—it will describe other ways to improve and enhance your skin's healthy and beauty using proven products, at home, simply and effectively.

What are Peels? How do I know what to get?

This might be the most important paragraph of the entire book, so read and go slow and buy carefully.

"Peels" are products with alpha hydroxy or glycolic acids—and sometimes other types of acids—that have been used for years by dermatologists and skin care profession-als and are designed to penetrate the layers of your skin and make significant changes in the tone and texture of your skin. Some Peels are too strong for home use and you should not ever attempt using them—even though you may find them on the internet! For instance—do not **EVER** attempt TCA Peels—those are so strong you can scar or disfigure yourself. Only a qualified doctor should work with those. We're not kidding—follow the careful advice we give in *The Skin Regime* and use the recommended Peels from compa-nies that we discuss in this book or on TheSkinRegime.com website. If you follow our instructions, you will be absolutely fine. Millions of people have discovered this and there are many safe at-home Peels—as long as you know and under-stand what you are getting.

Want to see some un-touched up before and after photos of women using at-home peels exactly like the ones written about it this book? Visit TheSkinRegime.com

These things called Peels—does that mean my skin will actually *Peel*?

Not always, not if you stick to the glycolic-acid peels we discuss here. You may get redness and some flaking—and perhaps a teensy bit of peeling at the stronger levels—but home-based products called Peels are not really peeling off your skin. Well, it is, but you can't often see it—it is happening in a very small, almost invisible way. Your skin is reacting to the Peel (you'll feel it somewhat and see it) and the skin cells are probably washing or sloughing off all day—so other than a bit of flaking, you might not see too much.

Okay, so where do I find Peels?

This is an incredibly important question.

The answer? Everywhere—all over the internet.

And that is a **big** problem, because there is a lot of stuff out there that is either no good or downright harmful. And there are the phonies and frauds and all that.

Don't push it—start with the widely-available and reputable lower-strength Peels. Your skin will build up tolerance for stronger preparations, you will get nice results. Or you may be perfectly happy with the results you get staying on the lower-strength Peels!

That is why TheSkinRegime.com has a continually-updating list of the best places to find the right Peels for you.

The best way to start is with a mild Peel you can find in the department store or at Sephora (or on Sephora.com). In department stores, at the well-known Clinique makeup counters, you can get their good starter-strength glycolic acid peel, called Radience Peel—several weeks worth for a decent price. (If you check online, you might be able to get Clinique products for less cost than the department store.) The Clinique kit comes with several mild Peels and if you do all of them over the course of a few weeks—you should see nice skin improvement. Almost everyone can tolerate those mild peels.

"Nice skin improvement" is what I wrote—I did <u>not</u> write "great improvement," and I did not write "superb improvement." Mild Peels can't give you a lot of change—and they are a great place to start. They will not only show you how it feels, but also how incredibly easy it is to do this. For better-than-"nice" improvement, you will probably need to move up to stronger preparations.

Sephora stores (and their online site) offer several companies that also produce low-level peels. See if you can get a sample or two instead of buying an entire peel kit.

On TheSkinRegime.com, we list other companies you can call to discuss your skin type and needs—and maybe get low-cost samples of the Peels they offer. (Tell them you read about it at The Skin Regime and put a smile in your voice—can't hurt!)

Always start with a lower strength Peel—generally this will be labeled as around 30% glycolic acid, although some Peels at 30% are stronger than another's 30%. Why would one be different from another? It has to do with how it is prepared, and other ingredients put in the formulation.

So even if you think you have tough skin, start with lower strength from these reputable companies and work your way up to stronger percentages of glycolic acid—your skin will most likely build tolerance and you will have almost no risk of anything going wrong.

Even if you don't use up all of a low-strength Peel formula and find you want stronger Peels, you can save and use the lower-strength Peels later in the Maintenance phase of *The Skin Regime* (read on).

> Disclaimer: Lawyers say we have to remind you that you do everything at your own risk, The Skin Regime doesn't assume liability, we can't guarantee that everyone else in the world is honest or that something might not go wrong with one of the products and all that.
> You know how it is....

The secret ingredient in Peels: Glycolic Acid (which is a part of the Alpha Hydroxy acid family). You can read all about the safety and efficacy of alpha hydroxy acid on respectable medical and informational websites if you want more evidence of it's safety and effectiveness. We list some of those sites—like the American Dermatology Association—on TheSkinRegime.com.

The nice thing about starting with lower-strength products from Clinique or Sephora and other reputable companies—if you don't like something, or have any issues at all, you can most likely get a full refund!

Once you are certain you are ready for stronger Peels, visit TheSkinRegime.com for resources of reputable places to find them. Talk to the representatives at these companies and discuss your skin type—they will be able to tell you what strength to try next—and maybe even have sample sizes.

You can't get stronger glycolic Peel preparations in stores—not yet, anyway. Why? Well, as I explained in Part One, companies just don't want to deal with all the questions. By keeping the Peels relatively mild—they are far less likely to get calls from people wondering why their skin is slightly red or flaking, etc.—normal reactions in stronger, more effective Peels.

The important thing is –DO NOT just buy any old Peel on the internet—you might be buying false or harmful products. TheSkinRegime.com has a continually-updating list of companies that are known to us.

Whatever glycolic preparation you have decided to start with—the instructions in this book will be the same for all of them—how to test and prepare your skin, and the right way to do it.

And much more than that! Keep reading.

Using Peels and other products

Stop using all your other skin-care products, with one exception: If you have a favorite eye cream, you may continue using it around the eyes, but avoid perfumed products. _Do NOT use any other products during The Skin Regime, as this can cause an adverse reaction_. Use only the Peels and products discussed in _The Skin Regime_—you'll have everything you need.

Just set aside all your toners, astringents, moisturizers, creams and other products that aren't really working for you anyway. You will probably never want return to those old products, but because you probably hate to throw away stuff—especially if you haven't used it all up—just put them away for now. You'll feel better about tossing them out later when you attain your beautiful skin and see for yourself that those other products were pretty useless.

Testing products

Anything you buy for your skin always says, "test before using." This is a very important step and it is very easy.

A day or so before you plan to begin _The Skin Regime_, test a product by applying some to a small patch on the inside of your arm, near the crook of the elbow, and another behind and under an ear. Try a different product on each of three days. You will know within 24 hours if you have allergies or other issues with a product.

How to know if a Peel is not right for you

It is NORMAL for the skin to turn red or feel a temporary stinging, itching or burning sensation when doing the Peels. It is NORMAL for the skin to peel a little or flake for a day or two (or more) after a Peel. That is what a peel is all about. HOWEVER, it is *not normal* to have a severe reaction, or swelling, or sensations that last more than a few minutes. Use your common sense, pay attention to what this book teaches you, and you'll know if *The Skin Regime* is working properly.

If a Peel is too strong for me, what do I do?

If you have really sensitive skin—or suspect you do—use products in the most mild strengths. You can always step up to stronger preparations after your skin starts to improve, adapt, and build a tolerance (tolerance is a good thing to expect). However, if you have an extreme reaction to any product, discontinue using it.

There are going to be some people who simply can't tolerate alpha hydroxyl acids. Some people can't eat peanuts—you never know how your body is going to respond to something until you try it. That is why you simply must test something—not on your face—before applying it on your face.

When should I do a Peel?

We suggest late afternoon or early evening, on a night you will just be hanging around your home. Your skin may turn pink or flushed in the hour or so following the Peel, and you may prefer not to go out that evening (although some people love the pink glow it can give you). Doing the Peel in the evening will give your skin time to calm down overnight.

DO NOT DO A PEEL in the week leading up to a big event like a wedding or important date—unless you don't mind that your skin may be peeling and flaking like it would after a mild sunburn. Your skin might *not* react that way, but why take the chance? Choose your timing to work with your plans for the "boot camp" weeks—the weeks that you will be regenerating new skin. Once you are on Maintenance, this will not be an issue, as your skin will always look superb.

> When used over a period of weeks, Peels described in *The Skin Regime* can give you nearly the same results as expensive laser or industrial-strength peels—unless you have deep scars, in which case you probably need the heavy-duty artillery. *The Skin Regime* is about gentler Peels over several weeks—not one big "peel." You won't have any "down time."

Exactly what is the time-frame for The Skin Regime?

If you have average skin with moderately troubling skin issues, you should see a noticeable difference in one to two weeks, and a big difference in six-to-twelve weeks. Each Peel needs seven to fourteen days in between, and each week, your skin gets closer to your glow-goal. Generally, after six Peels, you will have noticeably new-looking skin, which will continue to get better and better with simple Maintenance outlined in this book.

If you have very sensitive skin, the process *might* take a bit longer, as you will need to begin with less-potent products for your Peels and perhaps give your skin more time between Peels. As your skin builds up tolerance to the products, you can increase the strength—or you might find that you do just fine with more mild products.

If your skin is relatively tough, you may need to step up the strength of the products and do an extra Peel or two, perhaps for a total of seven or eight instead of six.

Exactly what should I expect in the beginning of The Skin Regime?

This is a very important question. Keep in mind that the goal is to gently slough off your old skin, regenerate new skin cells and nourish them. If you wanted to do this very quickly, you'd have to get a strong chemical or laser peel in the office of a plastic surgeon or cosmetic dermatologist. With those sorts of industrial-grade peels, you'd have many days of painful, oozing, peeling skin, and be unable to show your face during the healing time—you would have to take about two weeks of "downtime" at home to take care of the skin. The results of that sort of strong chemical peel can be uneven and take weeks for your skin and its pigment to smooth out. Plus, it costs thousands of dollars. *But even after going through all that*, you would still have to maintain your skin the same way *The Skin Regime* teaches you in order to keep your new skin looking great.

Over all, what *The Skin Regime* suggests is far more gentle. It takes more than a day, but it won't disrupt your life or budget.

However—and here is another important note—you might have some flaky skin lasting for a couple of days each time you do a Peel. Sometimes the flaky skin lasts for more than a couple of days—which is fine. That only means you really are getting a great reaction and sloughing off the bad old skin. Just to be on the safe side—since you really don't know how each Peel will turn out—you probably want to make sure you don't have someplace important to show your face in the days immediately following a Peel. It's possible you won't have too much peeling, but until you discover exactly how your skin reacts, you need to keep the transition-time in mind. Also, your response to each peel could vary—some Peels might elicit more of a reaction than others.

In many case, people love the way their skin looks in the days following a Peel: it can be rosy, smooth, glowing!

But until you know how your skin reacts to various strengths, you should take into account what is going on in your life a few days following a Peel.

Whenever possible, formulations for "sensitive skin" are chosen because they tend to be better for all skin types, and do not contain irritating perfumes.

Also, we often suggest buying "creams" and not "gels" or "ointments." Gels often have alcohol and are drying, and ointments are too gooey and oily. Creams go on smoothly, leaving little to no residue.

This is a matter of personal taste.

It is also important to know that it is *possible* your skin could go through a brief time of looking slightly worse before it looks better. In the beginning, you are introducing your skin to an entirely new process that goes deeper into the layers of skin—and unless they have been exposed to these products before, a lot of work is going to be happening. Your skin might react by becoming slightly irritated, even between Peels (we'll explain how to try to avoid that). If you have dark patches (melasma) on the skin, they may get slightly darker before they peel or fade away. Your acne may increase slightly. This adjustment period lasts a short time, and should not reappear ever again once your skin adapts and builds tolerance to the products while you maintain *The Skin Regime*.

The Products Needed for The Skin Regime:

Listed below are the mandatory products and a few suggested ones. *Be sure to note the strength and exact names of these products so you don't end up with the wrong formulation or preparation.*

Don't ever buy similar-sounding products! There are so many products out there that spell their names just a little differently, or claim they are "just as good as," a well-known product—and that is just not true! *The Skin Regime* lists the *exact* generic ingredients that are needed.

Would you buy tickets to see the *Rolling Spones* or *Alton John* and say, "That's close enough to the real guys." Don't think so. Therefore remember: Retinol is *not* Retin-A (treti-noin), and so on. Check the spelling, buy responsibly.

1. Rough washcloths. You want to buy cheap, rough cloths that will give you more exfoliating action (sloughing off dead skin cells). You can often find them bundled in packs of ten for a few dollars at places like Bed Bath and Beyond. Buy several. inexpensive dishtowels, cut into squares, are often perfect to use as rough cloths.

> Washcloths are a breeding ground for bacteria. Always use a clean, dry washcloth. Do not re-use a washcloth without first washing it after every use, preferable in hot soapy water. And keep in mind—go gently!

2. Dove Sensitive Skin Beauty Bar. That's right, good old Dove soap, low-priced and available everywhere. Do not buy the 'exfoliating' bar, buy the 'sensitive skin' formulation. If you can't find that in the drugstore or supermarket, the original-formula Dove soap is okay, but you are better off with the Sensitive Skin preparation. You can use Cetaphil cleanser as an alternative, also found in most drugstores.

3. Lubriderm Sensitive Skin Therapy Lotion. This is inexpensive and found in most drugstore chains and many supermarkets. You can use it on your face, around your eyes if you wish, on your body. However, it is not oil-free and that means it could block pores. If you have oily skin, get a non-blocking oil-free moisturizer such as Neutrogena Oil Free moisturizer or Aveeno Oil Free, or CeraVe—which makes an

oil-free moisturizer with broad-spectrum sun protection as well.

Glycolic Acid sounds scary, but is used in formulations in hundreds of products, even over-the-counter preparations. It is a category of alpha hydroxy acids (AHA) that are fruit-acid derivatives. The difference is that most cosmetic-company products are not strong enough to give you real results.

4. Glycolic Acid Solutions. Resources on where to find these peels are all over the web—be sure you get a reputable solution from a reputable company. Strength can vary. One company may sell a buffered 20% solution with a different ph-level, which could make it stronger than other solutions. Ask for guidance from any company you purchase from. At TheSkinRegime.com, we update a list of appropriate places to get Peels.

5. Plain rubbing alcohol from the drugstore. This will be used to prep the skin for the peel. If your Peel comes with a "pre-peel" preparation, you can use that, but many do not.

IF YOU HAVE SENSITIVE SKIN, start with a glycolic solution of, usually around 20%. You can always upgrade to stronger solutions. **IF YOU ARE SURE YOU HAVE VERY TOUGH SKIN**, then you will upgrade to a glycolic solution of around 40% or more, depending on your skin and the company you are using. Start low—you can always upgrade or downgrade strength. And don't purchase anything OTHER than AHA or glycolic acid solutions—there are strong and harmful chemicals (with different names) out there but those can burn your skin and should ONLY be used under physician guidance.

 An important note about sunscreen:

Yeah, we've been over this already, but it is so important, we must say it again. The sun is the single worst enemy to your skin. You have to protect your skin more than ever once you expose your new, fresh, glowing skin to the outdoors. If you are going to be exposed to the sun more than a couple of minutes, you must use sunscreen.

BUT SOME sunscreens might make you break out! So look for non-comedogenic screens, if possible, or get those we suggest on TheSkinRegime.com

Everyone is different, some people don't react to some sunscreens, others do.

Experiment with some from the drugstore—just make sure they offer the ingredients for full-spectrum protection, not just partial ray blocking.

For broad-spectrum light protection, you want to look for the words *zinc oxide* and/or *titanium dioxide* in the ingredients list of sunblocks. Those sound like ingredients from a nuclear reactor, but no—they are "inert," meaning—NOT ABSORBED into the skin. Therefore, they have no carcinogenic properties. Completely safe protection.

Those are the basic necessities for *The Skin Regime*. The following list has some other items you might find very useful:

1. <u>Benzoyl Peroxide 10% cream</u>. Available over-the-counter in most drugstores and supermarkets. We like Clearasil's cream (invisible formulation). You'll want this if you still get zits. If you have a zit you want to zap, put a little of this cream right on the little bugger as your last step of your evening. Don't use it on your entire face during *The Skin Regime*—it is too strong to use in combination with all the other products at the same time—too much is overkill and can cause irritation.

2. <u>Antibacterial cream</u> with "pain relief." Sometimes, especially early in *The Skin Regime*, your skin might get itchy and irritated, particularly around the corners of your nose and lips. In most drugstores, you can find an antibacterial cream with a formulation that sort of "numbs" the skin and relieves that irritation, as well as helps to prevent the irritation from getting worse. The one you want contains the active ingredient called *pramoxine HCl*. You'll find it in the drugstore aisle by the name of Bacitracin or Neosporin. Use just on the spots that feel irritated.

3. <u>Fish Oil</u>. Fish oil is one of the best all-around products for good health and good skin. Be sure you consult with a knowledgeable health-food store clerk about the best kinds. A good fish oil tablet will not have any fishy aftertaste. Check TheSkinRegime.com for lists of our favorite products.

4. <u>Vitamins</u>. Taking good care of your body with exercise and healthy food works wonderfully with *The Skin Regime*, but that is an entirely other book, isn't it? Meanwhile, try to make sure you are getting the proper vitamins, minerals, iron, calcium. A good daily multi-vitamin is really a must for everyone.

5. <u>Facial scrubs.</u> We strongly suggest you DO NOT use any exfoliating scrubs until a few weeks into the plan, and then only to help remove dead skin cells. And only if your skin is not irritated. A rough washcloth should do all the exfoliation you need if you are peeling. But if you feel you need a bit extra to remove flaking and dead skin cells, try squeezing a bit of gentle and non-perfumed facial scrub onto the washcloth—and keep the key word in mind: GENTLE.

> You may notice there are no "toners" or astringents in *The Skin Regime*. You don't need them and shouldn't want them. Many contain some alcohol and dries out the skin. Toners are often unnecessary – skip them.

6. <u>Large cotton balls or squares</u>. We like to use these to apply the glycolic acid, but you may find another method—such as simply using your fingers—works best for you.

7. <u>Disposable gloves</u> or other clean gloves. We suggest gloves because sometimes glycolic acid makes nail polish turn a bit dull if it comes in contact with it. So be careful not to get it on your nail polish (if you wear it), or put on some gloves—just make sure your hands and gloves are clean. Most major drugstores sell inexpensive boxes of fifty or more disposable gloves made of latex or another material (some people have latex allergies).

What you DO NOT want: You don't want to use any of the stuff you were using before. We mean *stop*.

Completely. No toners, no gels, no lotions, no creams—nothing except *maybe* your favorite eye-moisturizer as we mentioned before. Put everything else away or give it away.

An important note about self-tanning creams and lotions. They can bring out skin discoloration on some people. That seems *so* unfair, doesn't it? We can't go in the sun, we can't go to tanning salons, we can't use self-tanners? Good thing having a tan is not important to looking great! The color of a person's skin never has defined beauty—one can be beautiful with pale white or ebony skin. *Great skin* is what makes you look great. Nicole Kidman has always protected her skin, and no one is complaining about her lack of a tan.

In fact, people with perpetual tans are kind of like people puffing on cigarettes: We don't think smoking is so cool anymore—we think, "Whoa, working on getting cancer, girlfriend?"

So, if self-tanners don't work for you but you really want a "sun glow," reach for a good makeup bronzer.

Let's get to it! You have assembled all your necessary products and you're eager to get going on your new skin. Your chosen day has arrived and you're ready to go. We'll tell you again: Don't overdo it, be patient. If you rush *The Skin Regime*, you might mess it up by over-irritating your skin—then you'll have to stop and wait to get back on track. Be patient—your gorgeous new skin will start appearing very soon.

An important note to TEENAGERS!

Teenagers—you have special skin. It is still growing and going through changes and you probably hate your skin because, if you are a typical teen, you have acne.

If your acne is moderate, you can benefit a lot from following *The Skin Regime*—but please do so with your parents' knowledge and consent.

AND FOLLOW THE DIRECTIONS EXACTLY.

Do NOT think, "Oh, but *my* skin is special. I have *more* acne than all those really old people reading this book, who are, like, 34 or something like that. So I have to do *The Skin Regime* differently. I need to use *more*, do *more* Peels, and scrub really *harder* to exfoliate my skin."

No. No no no no no.

In fact, doing more can cause inflammation and damage and make matters worse. More does NOT mean "better."

If you have a high fever, do you take "more" aspirin instead of just two? No, because more aspirin or *ibuprofen* or *acetaminophen* (the stuff in Advil and Tylenol) can damage your liver. Two of fever-reducing pills will help you and bring down your fever, where as "more" can send you to the hospital.

Following *The Skin Regime* correctly will help you. Doing "more" is unlikely to send you to the hospital, but it is not good for your skin, either.

STARTING THE SKIN REGIME

The Peel

You have chosen the perfect time—most likely late afternoon or early evening. You have done your tests, and you have your Peel products ready.

Follow these incredibly simple steps.

1. Wash your face and neck thoroughly with Dove and your rough washcloth. Give your skin a moderately firm but gentle scrubbing with the washcloth. The idea is to gently exfoliate dead skin cells and have the cleanest skin possible for the products you are about to apply.

2. Go over your face with a cotton ball or square with the rubbing alcohol or peel-prep. Get it good, the idea is to strip your face of oils and other soap or residue which can prevent the Peel from interacting properly with your skin.

2. Let your skin dry completely, then apply your *glycolic acid* Peel on your face and neck with an absorbent tissue or cotton balls or squares. (Again, if you wear nail polish, you might want to avoid getting the glycolic acid on your nails as it might make some polish dull).

Be sure to extend Peel formulas below your jaw line and onto your neck, "feathering" (lightly extending some product) down toward the collarbone. This will create an even transition of skin tone and texture.

THE WAY TO APPLY: <u>Make sure there is no dripping</u>, as you don't want any solution to drip in the eye!

Work quickly, and start on the cheeks, forehead and neck, feathering down to the collarbone. Don't forget above the upper lip (but do not apply directly to the lips). Lastly, give a quick swipe under the eyes, keeping a good distance from the lower lid (be very careful so the product does not get in the eyes! If it does, flush eyes completely with cool water and start over).

Avoid applying to the very corners of the nose and mouth. If you're like most people you won't pay close attention to this advice, and therefore those areas will likely show irritation. Don't sweat it, it isn't going to kill you—but do at least *try* to avoid those areas.

The *glycolic acid* Peel may itch or sting. That is fine, it is supposed to. Try to leave it on as long as you can tolerate it, but NO LONGER THAN A FEW MINUTES. Read the instructions or info that comes with your product for what is appropriate.

3. After no longer than a few minutes, wash off gently with your recommended soap.

After this *glycolic acid* phase of the Peel, your skin may look very pink or flushed, as if you have a slight sunburn. That is normal and expected. Your skin may continue to feel itchy or stinging for a little while after you wash it off, but that sensation will disappear in a few minutes.

4. Immediately after washing, moisturize your skin thoroughly with your recommended moisturizer.

And that is all there is to *The Skin Regime*! Can you believe how easy that was? You have just begun your easy road to amazing skin.

You may wish to apply your favorite eye-cream—or simply use some moisturizer as your eye-cream or under the eyes or on other dry-feeling spots.

If you have a zit, dab a little of the *benzoyl peroxide* on it (optional).

If you have any lingering tingling or itchy spots after the Peel, dab on some of the antibiotic cream that contains *pramoxine HCl* (optional).

You're done for now. Sleep tight and see you in the morning!

After The Peel: The Evening and Morning Skin Regime

It is normal if your skin still appears a little flushed or perhaps feeling a little "tight" or dry after doing the Peel the night before. It might look a LOT flushed and slightly irritated. Or maybe it just looks pretty much as always. These results fine and normal.

What you will do for the next several mornings and evenings is so simple, you aren't going to believe it. Here it is:

1. Every morning and evening after the Peel, wash gently with your soap.

2. Apply your moisturizer—and as we noted, any of our recommended moisturizers make a fine around-the-eye cream as well.

3. If you will be outside and your moisturizer has no sunscreen in it, apply a moisturizing sunscreen.

4. If you have a zit, apply a dab of *benzoyl peroxide* on top of it in the evening.

This is all you need to do, almost *every day* for the rest of your life unless you are dealing with stubborn issues like dark spots and fine lines (we cover this in the following chapters).

After applying your moisturizer, you are free to apply any makeup you wish. We suggest oil-free, non-comedogenic (non-pore blocking) makeups.

Because your skin will begin to change, your old makeup foundation may begin misbehaving within a few days or so. If you use dry or matte bases, or powdered bases, you'll probably find it may just be too dry.

When your skin begins to change, you may wish to experiment with more moisturizing bases—or you may stop needing or wanting foundation altogether.

We will discuss more about the best makeup for your new skin in Part Four of this book.

More Peels with The Skin Regime (for a total of six):

Every seven to fourteen days you will choose an evening when you are <u>not irritated and not peeling or flaking.</u> Then REPEAT THE PEEL as described above.

NEVER do a peel sooner than seven days, and try not to wait longer than fourteen days between Peels. You want to do a <u>total of six Peels.</u>

In the seven to fourteen days between peels, you will simply wash and moisturize and use sunscreen or *benzoyl peroxide* as needed.

And each week, after each subsequent peel, more glowing and radiant skin will emerge.

Here are some common questions and answers:

The Peels are working but I don't always have the same amount of peeling and flaking with each Peel. What is going on?

If, after a few days of a peel, you're getting some peeling and flaking—a little or a lot—everything is going great. You can't really predict how your skin will react to each progressive Peel because your skin is changing during this time. Some people peel and flake a lot after their first Peel, some not until after the second or third Peel. Some never really have peeling that can be seen by the naked eye. Make your adjustments as described below, depending on how your skin is progressing throughout the Regime.

What if I am not peeling or flaking, an no redness—nothing—even after two or three full Peels?

What, do you have skin made of asbestos? No, just kidding. Okay, if you really don't think the lower-strength preparations are doing a thing, you can step up to stronger percentages of some of the products. If you are using a low percentage *glycolic acid peel*, try the next step up with your chosen Peel product. Again, TheSkinRegime.com maintains a frequently-updated list of tried-and-true companies you can call to discuss your needs.

> Keep in mind this is all about *exfoliation*, not irritation! Back off when the skin starts to get irritated. Be patient!

And one more thing you can try if the Peeling is going too slowly: Apply a very low glycolic-acid skin lotion in the evenings between Peels to boost the skin's exfoliation power (usually a lotion with 8%-15% percent *glycolic* or *AHA acid*—recommended brands are listed on TheSkinRegime.com. Some of the brands can be found in the drugstore, some must be ordered from special peel-production sites.

KEEP IN MIND that many people have no discernable (to the naked eye) peeling or flaking of the skin. That does NOT mean nothing is happening. Much is happening on the cellular level, where your skin is renewing. You will notice improvement in your skin with The Regime, you might just not notice it happening in the way of peeling and flaking.

After you have stepped up to higher-level *glycolic acid* Peels during the Regime, be sure to give yourself <u>at least</u> seven days in between Peels. Don't rush it, it will happen.

What if my skin is peeling too much or is too irritated after a Peel?

Use common sense and stop everything for a few days—except moisturizer. Then, you can start up on the products when things calm down. If you have over-sensitive skin, you probably need to downgrade your product percentages. Switch to the lowest level of glycolic solutions for the Peels.

If your skin is still too irritated after taking several days for a break, you probably have extremely sensitive skin and should consult a dermatologist before continuing.

What if I get a few zits?

Following the advice of *The Skin Regime* will help a lot with acne, but not for severe or cystic acne. If it is a matter of a few overall breakouts or even just one or two zits, this is where the *benzoyl peroxide* comes in handy. Dab some of it on the zit every evening. It helps dry it up. And keep in mind that you may have a couple of weeks with a few extra pimples when you begin *The Skin Regime*, as your skin is "throwing out" lots of gunk, removing clogs and dead skin layers, and working to create new skin.

What if my dark spots don't completely fade away?

If you have uneven skin tone or melasma, a lot of it—or perhaps all of it—will fade after six Peels as described with *The Skin Regime*. If you have some lingering issues, keep reading—we have the answers in the next chapter!

After Six Peels:

> Instead of a maintenance Peel every few weeks after your series of six, you might like to experiment by applying a glycolic lotion every week or so, perhaps for one or two evenings. This might be just enough to keep your skin in tip-top shape and prevent ever needing to do a full Peel with stronger glycolic again.
> Your skin will be your guide.

After you have Peeled for a total of six Peels—roughly six to twelve weeks for most everyone (8 at most)—your skin should be greatly improved and glowing. You're done!

Now you need to leave "boot camp" and stop all Peels. You don't want to overdo it and harm your new skin. Let it glow, enjoy your new skin. Your new maintenance regime (next chapter) will help your skin grow increasingly more beautiful over the months and years ahead.

Should I ever do a Peel again, after going on Maintenance?

Every few weeks after your last Peel (the last of six total), you may wish to do one Peel as maintenance just to keep your skin fresh. Even without Peels, your skin will continue to get better and better.

In a year or so, you may wish to repeat the entire *Regime*, but most likely you will find your skin is doing fine with a Peel every eight weeks or so. Just be sure not to overdo it—listen to your skin.

Will *The Skin Regime* be the same for the rest of my life?

Is your butt the same at age sixteen as thirty-six? Is your hair the same? Is winter the same as summer?

No way around it, you will go through many phases in life such as hormonal changes—even if you are a guy—and you need to adapt your skin care to your life circumstance. You may find that you need stronger glycolic percentages to get a Peel, or perhaps less. You may develop dark patches after hormone changes—like after having children, or hitting menopause. And extreme weather changes means you have to adapt what you are doing for your face. Chlorine or salt water can make you more sensitive to your products, so you need to keep your lifestyle in mind, too. Winter can be irritating and drying, so you may want to treat your skin as "sensitive" during cold seasons. *Adapt* is the key word. And we keep saying it: Listen to your skin.

> You might like to know that products with glycolic acid often have a bitter taste. Therefore, don't apply any if you plan to be getting kissy-face with anyone that night… or day.

As time goes on, you will discover exactly what works for you and what needs to be updated as your body and skin changes. If a medical problem comes up, get to a good dermatologist (one that specializes on cosmetic dermatology).

The Skin Regime will also update information on the web and in print as science invents newer, better products that work—and we mean *really* work, not just the blathering baloney stuff that wastes our time and money.

Great, affordable, home-based skin care is not only possible, it will get even better as time goes on. Keep checking in with us at TheSkinRegime.com.

As mentioned at the beginning of this section, if you decided Peels aren't for you, read on to Maintenance and discover other ways to get great skin with great proven products, at home. Whether you do Peels or not—it is an important section for creating and continuing your skin care.

PART THREE

Maintenance for Your
New Skin with The Skin Regime

Whether or not you have followed previous *The Skin Regime* section on Peels—this is an important section for creating and continuing your skin care. You can get great skin by following the instructions here, or use the info to maintain the skin you now have post-Peels.

Beyond the Peels

Okay, you've done your series of six, or perhaps more, Peels. You can see an incredible difference and improvement in the look and quality of your skin.

Maybe that is all you need and want. Maybe you are done and will simply wish to continue maintaining your skin with a Peel every few weeks, and protection with sunscreen.

Or maybe you feel a few issues still need to be addressed. Perhaps there are some stubborn melasma spots. Or perhaps you are excited by what you have achieved, but you want to reach for even *better* skin.

Maybe you feel like a person who lost 50 pounds, sees how great her body looks in a sexy dress, and now wants to sculpt the muscles.

You can go for even more extraordinary skin, and this chapter, and the following chapters, will explain how to reach the next levels.

Prescription creams

Two of the miracle products we discuss here—again, there are no "secret" ingredients, we reveal all the truth—are, as of this writing, only available via prescription. These are *tretinoin* creams, and *hydroquinone 4%* creams.

You can show this book to your family physician and get a prescription for them, or visit a dermatologist for them, if you feel you want to try them. In some states, pharmacists can help you out. It should be fairly easy to get prescriptions for them—after all, these are not dangerous or controlled substances, but wonderfully beneficial products for the skin.

Why are these creams available only by prescription?

You know, it is so frustrating. You can buy truly dangerous items by the fistful on the shelves—even aspirin can kill you if you take too much—but a little dab of a face cream known to have fabulous benefits for almost every type of skin and minimal side effects? *Those* have to be kept under lock and key? Arggh!

In the case of *tretinoin*, this has more to do with politics and money. It is such a great product that certain pharmacies want to force you to have to purchase the product through them. As of this writing, the companies that make *tretinoin* are trying to get their product listed as non-prescription.

The benefits of *tretinoin* have been documented for decades—it helps with all kinds of skin issues including acne, fine lines, sun damage, and discoloration. *Tretinoin*-based preparations are often the first thing dermatologists suggest when a patient comes in for treatment.

What about hydroquinone? Isn't there controversy about the safety of that?

Yes, because some people have used this great chemical ingredient inappropriately. Hydroquinone is used to lighten dark patches on the skin. When used short-term, as directed, it is perfectly wonderful and safe as most FDA-approved medicines are.

Unfortunately, like any good medicine, some people abuse and overdose. As a result, there are questions about whether hydroquinone should be distributed to the public at all. That argument is similar to the painkiller controversy of recent years: Because some people abuse painkillers, does that mean people who need them shouldn't get them? It makes no sense.

People who use too much hydroquinone often do so because they are unhappy with their natural-born skin color. They use it all over their face and body, day after day and month after month to lighten their skin color a shade or two. This is very unwise, and possibly quite unhealthy. And worse—it is a sad commentary on how some people don't feel their naturally dark skin is attractive.

Do not worry about using hydroquinone-based products on the face for short-term use, as instructed in this book. It works, and once your irregularly-pigmented dark spots are gone, they stay gone—*unless you expose your skin to sunlight without protection*. You may need a touch up from time to time, but the quantities needed are extremely small and—as we noted before—probably a whole lot safer than eating most processed "food."

Keep in touch with TheSkinRegime.com for updates on new products that become available to the public and when or if prescription products become over-the-counter. Meanwhile, a good family doctor or dermatologist should be very open to giving you a prescription for a tube of *tretinoin* or hydroquinone if you tell them about *The Skin Regime* and why you want the creams. One tube of *tretinoin* should last you six months to a year! Same with *hydroquinone*.

...me reveals what <u>most</u> people can expect—not what ...gle individual on the planet might experience.

...s a really good Maintenance plan:

...ach night, while trying any of these Maintenance ...ucts, simply wash your face and let your skin dry thor-...nly—for least ten minutes. <u>Then take a really good look</u> <u>...evaluate what is going on</u>.

If you are irritated around the corners of your nose and ...outh and a few other places on the face, AVOID using any-...ing except moisturizer on those places. If you are irritated all ...ver, then use only moisturizer for a night or two until your ...kin calms down a bit.

"Listen" to your skin. Do not worry that taking off a cou-ple of evenings will slow down the progress or maintenance of your new skin—it won't.

As for that antibiotic cream we told you about earlier under "suggested products?" That is a great thing to apply if you have some itchy, irritated spots.

It is very common to get irritated at the corners of nose and mouth if you have accidentally applied the *tretinoin* or *glycolic acid* products there.

After a couple of months on Maintenance, you will prob-ably be ecstatic with the ongoing improvement of your skin. Keep it up, keep it simple, "listen" to your skin, and you will likely enjoy great skin for the rest of your life. It really is this easy.

Okay. Now let us talk about these products and why they are so great.

Tretinoin Cream .05%.

This is the Holy Grail of skin treatment and will be the single most important item that will help maintain your skin and take it to the next level of beauty.

As we said, it is available by prescription, marketed most commonly under the brand name <u>Retin-A</u>. You need to start using it gradually--until your skin gets used to it, it may cause some peeling and irritation, a lot like the Peels did.

IF YOU HAVE SENSITIVE SKIN, you might wish to start with a less-strong percentage of <u>Retin-A</u>, such as *tretinoin .025%.* You can always "upsize" the strengths later on.

> The tretinoin-based product "Tretin-X" has a reputation of being gentler for sensitive skin. Consider it as an alternative prescription to Retin-A.

PLEASE NOTE that very very little goes a very very long way with *tretinoin* cream. It comes in small tubes, but should last many months if you follow the instructions carefully.

Hydroquinone 4% cream.

Good-bye melasma patches!

This cream is available by prescription, as we noted. You can buy "fade creams" over-the-counter in drugstores and beauty stores that contain *hydroquinone 2%*, but they just aren't as effective as the 4%.

This cream is used on a short-term basis for skin discoloration—if you have no skin discoloration, skip it. In general, it should be used only on discolored skin patches—melasma—but if you have wide-spread discoloration, it can be used on the entire face.

Your dark patches should be vastly improved—or completely gone—in two to three months of using this cream. Stop using the *hydroquinone* and stay out of the sun, and you may never see those spots reappear!

Again, a little goes a very long way and do NOT use all over your body to lighten the skin!

How do I use tretinoin or hydroquinone creams?

First, read the information that comes with the products.

If you are using moisturizers containing Glycolic acid—stop for now—it will be too much.

Wash with your Dove soap at night, or other suggested cleaner, and wait for the skin to dry completely—at least ten minutes. Twenty minutes is even better. Then apply the *tretinoin* cream to your entire face, and feather it down below your jaw line and down a bit to your neck.

Do not worry about taking a few ni
turizer—you will not lose time gettin
Using an over-the-counter antibiotic c
should relieve any temporary irritation.

IMPORTANT: Use very very littl
Surprisingly little. An amount the size of a
your face and a little dab should disappear a
you begin to rub it in. A little goes a very long
more just wastes money. Keep away from ey
the glycolic acid, try to avoid the corners of yo
mouth.

After the *tretinoin* has set for at least twent
apply the hydroquinone ONLY on dark or discolore
of your skin (*apply directly on top of the tretinoin; do
your face again*).

One or both of the creams are irritating my skin—is t okay?

It is normal for *tretinoin*, and possibly *hydroquinone*, to cause some irritation when you first start using it. Just back off for a day or two, wait for the irritation to subside, and try again. Eventually, your skin should build up a tolerance and it will not be irritated, but instead start to look more and more amazing.

Of course, common sense is the rule. If you get a severe reaction—STOP. Not every product is for everybody. *The*

The Skin Regime works wonderfully for most hyper-pigmentation and melasma, but a really stubborn dark spot probably needs more than what you can do at home. <u>Keep in mind that for a couple of weeks during The Skin Regime, the dark spots may appear slightly darker before they peel or fade away</u>. This is normal and expected.

If your melasma returns at some point in the future, you may begin a few weeks of using *hydroquinone* on the spots again. But if you use sunscreen and continue using *tretinoin*—you will likely not have it reappear.

If, after a couple of months on Maintenance with *The Skin Regime*, you still have some really stubborn dark spots that are fading but refuse to completely disappear, consider a consult with a cosmetic dermatologist. They may be able to use some laser technology on those spots. The new Fraxel lasers are remarkable, and the procedure is done quickly, in the office, with little or no down-time. Lasers can remove all kinds of scars and improve severe skin issues dramatically.

 Some people might get the idea that if *The Skin Regime* works so well on the face, wouldn't it be a great idea to use it all over the body for all-over fabulous skin? DUMB. Don't do it. In fact, it can be dangerous. These are great products when used on the face—a relatively small area of your body—but can possibly be toxic when spread all over your body.

Body lotions with glycolic acid that contain low percentages (usually 4%-8%) can be used with regularity over the body, as can sunscreens—but don't use prescription items all over without consulting your dermatologist.

Think about it: Your skin absorbs many types of medicines and chemicals. When used only on the face and neck area, you're fine, but you must not make the potentially dangerous mistake of slathering this stuff everywhere. Keep in mind: Two aspirin is wonderful and beneficial for your headache. But a whole bottle of aspirin is very dangerous to you. Same with nearly any product you use, such as vitamins (or even chocolate!).

Consider all cosmeceuticals as medicines and use them appropriately, the way they are designed to be used.

PART FOUR

Enjoying Your New Skin:
Makeup and More

Now you have great, glowing new skin and know the simple steps to maintain it.

You want to show it off! How?

Perhaps you used makeup foundation to hide your flaws before you acquired your new skin, or perhaps you used too much eye makeup to distract attention from your skin.

With your new skin, you won't need to hide anymore, but you may want to enhance, to get the most from the "canvas" of your face and your new-found natural beauty.

After *The Skin Regime*, the quality of your skin will have changed for the better and your old foundation may be completely wrong for you now.

Time to have fun! Experiment with new makeup! Or try going bare-skinned. Just put on your moisturizer or sunscreen and go! *Naked skin is sexy.*

We will share our personal opinions as well a some great tips for makeup. There are tons of books and websites about makeup and makeovers, so we'll just stick to the tried-and-true basics that really work.

Makeup is a very personal preference and taste, and is as unique for each person as hairstyle, perfume, clothing and accessory choices. Whatever works for you—go for it.

Test before you buy.

> Be sure to use the disposable makeup sponges, cotton swaps and tissues provided at testing counters. Be wise and ask for clean testers.

Never buy any makeup you can't test on your skin—the colors always look different on you than they do behind plastic packaging or color swatches. So if there are no testers in the drugstore—skip it. Try going to stores like Sephora or department store makeup counters where you can experiment hands-on with testers.

Right off the bat, we'll say we're not generally a fan of expensive department store makeup because they are over-priced and often over-perfumed. Some can block your pores or irritate you. You can get nearly identical preparations with good drugstore brands like Revlon and L'Oreal—but you may not be able to test the colors. Sometimes, when a new color series comes out, there will be testers in the larger drugstores. Spring and Fall is a good time to find those new lines.

After you have found some colors you like, go to a window and look at yourself in natural light—don't depend only on in-store lighting. Even if they have lamps at the counters, it is not the same as natural light. If there is no natural light within a reasonable distance and you still believe the makeup is a good match for you, ask the salesperson if they will accept a return "just in case" the makeup ends up looking too orange or pink, or if you have any other issue with it at home. Most major brands and major drug and department stores will allow full returns with your proof of purchase.

Foundation

One exception to our overall aversion to department store brands is Clinique. We think they make very good makeup products that are reasonably priced (compared to the prices of some other department store brands). They have a lot of different foundations for different skin types, but our personal favorites have moisturizing bases and a bit of "glow," in their formulations. Their "Supermoisture" foundations are very moisturizing (maybe too much for some people), and their "Almost Makeup" is very light and has an SPF of 15—sunscreen protection is always a plus. You may prefer an oil-free preparation. They have good advisors.

Another thing you can try: Buy a heavier foundation and depending on how much color and coverage you want, you can mix up your own formula by adding some of your sunscreen or moisturizer. This will allow you to create your own "sheer tint" or "medium tint" formulation. This trick works very well with nearly all makeup bases.

With all the new foundations on the market, there is no excuse to have anything that looks heavy or cakey. Certainly not with your new, great skin! There are very light preparations and concealers that deposit a lot of color without a thick or "makeup-y" feel on your skin.

Nice salespeople at makeup counters are often happy to give you a makeover. But remember, their job is to convince you to buy as much makeup as possible. Don't be intimidated, don't feel obligated. Buy what you feel really works for you, and don't be afraid to walk over to a competitor's counter and get an entirely different opinion.

Matte preparations never really look natural, and can actually make the skin look dry or chalky—avoid those. If you get an oily nose or forehead and like to apply powders, we suggest first blotting the oil with a tissue or towel and then apply just the slightest amount of fine powder to absorb the rest. Using a soft, fluffy brush to apply powder gives a more natural look.

A lot of dermatologists are very enthusiastic about the new "mineral" make-ups—but it is a matter of personal taste. A good place to experiment with them is at your local Sephora store.

Blushers, Tints, Cheek Stains and Bronzers

Maybe you don't even need a foundation—maybe you just need a hint of color like you can get in a blush or a bronzer. Blush powders may look dry on your new, dewy skin. Cream blush goes on much smoother and blends better. Apply directly on cheekbones, and a dab around the temples (blending toward the forehead). A faint hint on the chin, perhaps.

Tints and cheek stains are often super-saturated with color and can be very tricky to work with. They can "stain" the skin by depositing too much color in one spot that won't blend easily and then the only way to remove that too-much color is to wash your face and start all over (and some of the stains don't even come off with one wash!)

Bronzers also provide color. Find one that works for you.

If you love the color of your powder-blush or powder-bronzer and don't want to give it up, but want a more natural look, try applying it to your cheekbones then blending with a dab of your moisturizer.

Whichever sort of blush product you choose to use, it should go right on top of your foundation. The biggest secret of getting it all to look natural on your face is BLENDING. Sometimes a small extra dab of moisturizer or sunscreen will help blend the products and keep it all looking smooth.

Eyes and Eyebrows

Don't over-tweeze your eyebrows—you'll regret it at some point. Keep them neat and full to accent your eyes. A small bit of hair gel or hair spray brushed on will keep them in place. (Some hair products "flake" on the eyebrows. Sephora and other brands have clear or tinted products that are made specifically to keep the eyebrows in place, and they don't flake).

Here is a big secret: You don't need special product to remove eye makeup. It is very important to completely remove eye makeup every evening, and using simple, inexpensive mineral oil as your first step before cleansing does a good job and will not irritate the eyes (mineral oil can be found in supermarkets or drugstores often under "laxatives," because it is also used to lubricate the intestines). In fact, some "eye makeup remover" is simply a mix of mineral oil and witch hazel or other cleanser containing alcohol, which can irritate or dry your eyes. Good old-fashioned, inexpensive Pond's Cold Cream is a mineral-oil based cream that works well, too.

The best way to apply mineral oil is with a cotton ball. Don't worry if some of it gets in your eyes, it won't hurt them.

As for eye shadows and such: Again, this is a personal decision on how much to use. Our tastes runs to neutral and natural colors used to *enhance*, not to hide or mask the eyes. Go very easy on eye color during the day, and a bit more dramatic at night.

> The best makeup tip: BLEND!!!

Knowing exactly how to bring out your eyes is one of the best things you can learn to do for your face. This is where getting suggestions from good salespeople or a makeup artist can be helpful. Don't just take the advice of one person—try a few different opinions. Tell them what your tastes are. You needn't buy the products they push on you—remember, they should be helping you, not coercing you to purchase.

In general, soft eyeliner pencils give a more natural look. Blending and smudging is key for a soft, natural look. Don't use too much under the eye, it "drags" your eyes down and makes them tired-looking instead of lifting up and looking upbeat and refreshed.

The older you get, the less "sparkle" or glittery look you want in your makeup, especially on your eyelids. Instead, use creamy matte colors and put subtle sparkle highlight just under the eyebrow and a small blended touch on the center of the lid.

Mascara is a pain—they all clump. No reason you should waste money on expensive ones—go with the drugstore brands. Maybelline's Great Lash has been around forever and is very reliable. To keep the mascara from getting too clumpy too soon, do not "pump" the wand—that pushes air inside the little tube. Swirl the mascara wand in the tube, then pull out.

The best way to avoid clumps and lumps is to use a round mascara brush and "twirl" the color on, then use a clean eyelash brush to smooth out any clumping before it dries. And be sure to replace mascara roughly every three months as it can breed bacteria.

Black mascara is often too harsh for anyone unless they have very dark hair—brown-black is often a better choice of mascara color.

> It is a good idea to keep your makeup closed and clean, less than a year old, and use clean brushes and sponges with clean hands before putting any on. Also best not to share brushes and sponges—and certainly do not share mascara!

What about dark circles under my eyes?

Don't be suckered into products that claim to eliminate dark circles. There is no cure for dark circles—yet—not even having plastic surgery. Sorry to tell you the truth, but there you have it. When a real cure comes out, we'll let you know.

Until then, there are ways to minimize and conceal dark circles or puffy eyes and reduce redness.

Here are some great ways to minimize and treat those issues:

1. Cool eye packs or eye masks. This feels great and works quickly and well to reduce puffiness and tired-looking eyes. You can get an inexpensive eye mask and keep it in the fridge. Or soak a washcloth in ice water, wring out and place over eyes.

As for under-eye concealers—be really careful with these. More often than not, you end up looking strange with pale circles that bring out every line. And many end up looking dry and cakey. Using moisturizer and a gentle application of some of your makeup base is often better.

If you haven't got time for that, try a very cold water splash over your eyes when you get up in the morning. Anything cold helps.

2. Get enough sleep.

3. Don't rub or scrub your eye area. Treat the area gently.

4. Stop smoking. Sunlight is the single worst thing for your skin, smoking is the second worst.

5. Get some exercise to get the blood flowing and encourage a healthy flush for the skin.

6. Gently massage your face with moisturizer to get the blood flowing better through the area.

7. Here is our best tip on how to perk up tired-looking eyes: Use a skin-toned (based on *your* skin tone) eyeliner or concealer or shadow *right under the lower lashes*, close to the lower lid—even go between the lashes. Go with a shade or two lighter than your skin color. The effect is immediate. Then apply your eye makeup as you normally would—or just keep the "nude" look.

What about my red eyeballs?

Stop rubbing them! If you have irritated eyes, use a soothing eyewash (available in drugstores. They come with an eye cup and go by names of Collyrium, or Bausch and Lomb Eye Relief Eyewash or OcuFresh). Try keeping this stuff in the fridge—the cold eyewash clears up red eyes almost instantly! And it feels so good.

During the day, use moisturizing eye drops for dry eyes. AVOID the use of "redness remover" drops and only use if all else fails. Why? These can actually be more drying and irritating and like a sugar rush, once they wear off, your eyes are redder than before—in some cases. We find eyewashes and lubricating drops work better for soothing and preventing dry, red eyes.

Lips

There are very simple ways to keep your lips soft, moist and looking great. The key is keeping them properly lubricated. But the problem is: "Which product to choose?"

Here again, one of the least expensive is the best. All those expensive lip products that make promises are unnecessary, and in some cases can do more harm than good. What we have found works best is the original formula of Blistex Medicated Lip Ointment. It is the one in the tube (the *ointment*, not the waxy stick balm) and found in nearly every drugstore and most supermarkets. The original formula is simply unbeatable.

Waxy lip balms or other preparations tend to make the lips feel moist *temporarily*, but Blistex really gets into the layers and does the trick. *Avoid products made with petroleum jelly* as the primary ingredient (Vaseline, for instance).

Petroleum jelly products mostly provide a temporary, non-effective moist feeling and do nothing to help cure dry lips.

Blistex ointment also makes a superb base for lipstick and doesn't feel waxy or gooey. And your hair won't stick to Blistex when the wind blows—if you have long hair, you know what we're talking about! Keep a tube handy and apply several times a day, and you'll lose those peeling chapped lips in a few days.

And those so-called "lip plumpers?" They irritate the lips and give you sensation of swelling, but they don't really work. Many of them can actually dry out your lips.

Avoid matte lipsticks and lip "stains," and the products that claim to last all day—they tend to be drying, not hydrating. Stick to moisturizing lipsticks and glosses (again, the major drugstore brands are super). For extra help and a smoother feel, apply your lip color right after you put on some Blistex.

And don't forget the sunscreen! If you'll be outside, choose a moisturizing lipstick or gloss with some sunscreen in it, or apply clear sunscreen before your color or after you have applied Blistex.

In the evening when you brush your teeth, brush your lips to exfoliate them—then apply Blistex as part of your Maintenance regime.

Smile!

The best way to give your skin an instant "lift" and glow is to develop the habit of maintaining a slight smile on your face. Watch your face in the mirror and see how just the smallest upturn pulls up your cheeks and adds beauty to your face. A smile is one of the simplest and most attractive things you can add to *The Skin Regime*.

Many of us walk around carrying our worrisome thoughts on our faces. It shows. We bet that even right now, your muscles are tense.

Take a breath and release the muscles of your forehead and jaws, allow your mouth to open slightly. You can feel it smooth out, can't you? And how quickly those muscles tense up again! Try to get in the habit of releasing those muscles during the day—it will not only reduce your inner stress, but help you create a smoother appearance as well.

Teeth.

And what happens when you open that mouth to smile? Are you showing your pearly whites or brown-tinged yellows? Okay, so maybe your teeth aren't technically part of your skin, but let's hit this subject anyway.

Drug-store whitening strips and gels do work—not as well as a dentist-office whitening treatment, but you can get noticeably whiter, cleaner-looking teeth with drugstore-brand whitening systems, like Rembrandt, or Crest strips.

And as long as we went there—sorta—let's put in a word about bad breath. Brush your teeth and gums well, and use a tongue scraper or brush your *tongue* thoroughly each night to help cut back on bad breath and germs that can harm your teeth and gums. Add in a mid-day brushing to keep things fresh.

Covering up with mints and sprays is very temporary. Especially if you have that coming-from-inside, ate-garlic-and-onions sort of breath. What works: Eat an apple. Eat some parsley. Either works pretty well.

PART FIVE

Beyond The Skin Regime: Fillers, Lasers, Lifts, Lipo and Meds, and Other Stuff

Aren't there products that provide a face-lift effect?

No.

But--?

No buts. Only phony baloney claims from products.

Honestly, there is no cream or product that lifts and tightens sagging skin or removes deep age wrinkles—you really need a reality check if you believe in a product that makes those claims.

The Skin Regime is going to give you gorgeous, glowing skin, but if you want a face-lift, you need a plastic surgeon. Surgery is the most expensive and drastic option but the results can be wonderful and long-lasting.

By "surgery" we mean everything from an eye lift, to lipo-suction on the neck and jaw-line, to a complete facelift. You can do a little, you can do a lot. We've all seen so many before-and-after jobs that look natural and can vastly improve deep wrinkles, remove fat deposits under the eyes, and smooth seriously scarred skin. And if the work of a plastic surgeon is really done well, you don't know you are seeing any "work done"—the client just looks *good*. It is a very personal choice and decision.

> You will need a plastic surgeon or cosmetic dermatolo-gist for laser treatments. Some intense treatments may require "down time" as your skin recovers. Look under "resources" at TheSkinRegime.com to see how to find appropriate board-certified doctors.

Of course, we've all seen the celebrities—and others—who have overdone it and look completely weird and fake—just more proof that being famous or rich doesn't auto-matically give you common sense or good taste. So if you decide on plastic surgery, go easy, choose a good surgeon and make sure he/she understands you want a natural look for enhancement. You do not want to end up resembling an extra-terrestrial!

There are so many choices—expensive and not-so-expensive—for improving the way you look. For scars and/or old acne pits, there are wonderful improvements that can be done with lasers on small areas, or entire facial resurfac-ing. Much of these can be done relatively painlessly in the doctor's office, not in a hospital.

What about needles?

For deep lines that run from the corners of your nose to your mouth, you can get injectable fillers given by a plastic surgeon or a cosmetic dermatologist skilled in the art of "fillers" with brand names such as Restylane or Juvederm.

If you have really thin lips, you might want injectables, too. Here again, you want to do have it done right, and not over-do it. The lips should match the face and subtle is better than too-much.

A little lip-liner and keeping your lips moist and conditioned might be all you need or want.

Botox. Ah, the glory of Botox—it is really good stuff. It works great on crow's feet around the eyes and some creases on the forehead—but here again, you want to go easy. Less is better than more. A good Botox treatment will not hinder emotional facial expression or your natural look, and it should <u>not</u> remove every line on your face. Having a "frozen" face is simply bizarre looking—instead of looking younger, you will look like someone who had "too much work done." And without the ability to show emotion, people might get strange "cues" from you. You can end up looking vacuous and vague.

With Botox, you have to get treatments every few months, as the effect wears off. And you don't want to bargain-shop for a doctor to do it—find a good cosmetic dermatologist or plastic surgeon with the proper training in the art of Botox injections. Like with anything else, there are good doctors and bad ones—a bad one can really mess you up and it can take months for the Botox to leave the spot that gets messed up.

Botox is also expensive, but the good news is that some competing products are going to be coming out that should allow for some price competition as well as a choice in similar products.

Bottom line: Get injectables if you want, just don't be an idiot about it.

Oral Meds?

There is pill for almost everything these days, right? Even things we never heard of—such as a pill for people whose legs are restless. Really?

And yet hair-thinning and cellulite remain as uncured as the common cold—don't fall for bogus pills that say they treat those conditions.

But severe acne sufferers have pills that <u>do</u> work. You'll need a good dermatologist to advise you about prescriptions for severe acne if it involves taking *isotretinoin* (such as Accutane or Sotret), or antibiotics. You must be monitored closely during the months you are on *isotretinoin*, and women must be on birth control—but for severe or cystic acne, it is truly a wonder drug, taken only for a few months and can cure severe acne for years or a lifetime.

I've got hair… but not where I want it.

If you have unwanted facial or body hair, laser hair removal is a great choice, and provides permanent hair removal after a few treatments. And let's just say it because you may have been suffering in silent embarrassment: Having hair around the nipples is not that uncommon, ladies. Get thee to a laser hair removal specialist. Believe us—the techs who do this stuff have seen it all.

Electrolysis is also permanent and effective, but is more painful and expensive than laser hair removal. However, it might be a better choice if you just have one or two stubborn strays. But because of the success of laser hair removal, it is getting harder and harder to find electrolysis technicians.

Bleaching instead of removing hair.

Thank heavens for the body-hair bleach creams made by Jolen and Sally Hansen and others which you can find in the drugstore—they work very nicely for a little dark peach fuzz on the face, belly, arms.

Quick tip: If using those bleaches make your skin "itch" when you put them on, try spraying some Solarcaine or Lanacane First Aid Spray (in drugstores) or other sunburn spray BEFORE putting on the bleaching cream--it should make it itch less. And do NOT exfoliate your skin before using the bleach—do it afterwards and be sure to follow with lots of moisturizer. If you have sensitive skin, use a sensitive-skin body-hair bleach formula.

What about cellulite?

Again, there are too many fraudulent claims and bogus products. The only way to *improve* the look of cellulite on the body is diet and exercise—but even then it will not completely disappear.

A little trick used by models and makeup artists: Using a little self-tanner on the legs can help to camouflage cellulite. It helps minimize the appearance of lots of little leg flaws—give it a try.

The simple hard truth is—there is not yet a cure for cellulite. But perhaps soon…

Not even liposuction?

Not even liposuction.

Liposuction can remove fat from just about anywhere—neck, face, under eyes, arms, legs, stomach, thighs—and thus improve the way those areas look. But the dimples and ripples of cellulite simply cannot be sucked away by lipo. Massage machines, creams, special machines and gadgets, pills, surgery, lasers—they don't work on cellulite.

Not yet anyway. We're sure they'll find a way to remove cellulite one day, but it just isn't here yet.

Sorry to be so cold about it, but *The Skin Regime* is committed to revealing the hard truths about products involving your skin and body, and this is one of those truths.

Don't shoot the messenger.

PART SIX

The Rest of Your Body: The Skin Regime for Elbows, Hands, Feet, Knees, Hair and All-Over Good Skin Care

It is so gratifying when you see how *The Skin Regime* works so simply and well for your face that you will want to apply some of what you learned to the rest of your skin.

But you can't do the exact same thing on your body or use the exact same products—the skin on your body requires different care and not all of the products designed for the face are appropriate for use on the body.

You should not use high percentages of *glycolic acid* or *tretinoin* in large quantities as we already explained in Part One of this book, and will repeat here again: These are great products when used on the face (a small area), but can possibly be toxic when spread all over your body. Think about it: Your skin absorbs medicines and chemicals and some part of those medicines can get into the bloodstream. When used only on the face/neck area, you're fine, but don't make the potentially dangerous mistake of slathering this stuff everywhere.

Having healthy skin starts with being healthy. Exercise, eat right, get appropriate rest, lower your stress, and take vitamins.

Let's start at the top and work our way down.

Hair

There seem to be more products for hair than there are for the face! Far too many choices and just as many price levels. But like other skincare products, you don't have to reach for expensive ones when cheaper products are just as good if not better.

Hair issues often parallel skin issues and you need to use just as much common sense in treating problems. If you have severe issues such as the sudden appearance of unusual thin or bald spots—sometimes called *alopecia*—you would consult a dermatologist. Rashes, cysts, moles, patches of scaly skin on the scalp—they require medical attention and a dermatologist is the right doctor for the job.

Most hair-loss commercials are designed for men, and most advertised products are totally bogus. There are safe and proven products to help (not cure) some thinning hair issues, such as topically-applied solutions that contain *minoxidil*, known more commonly by the product name of Rogaine. You can buy *minoxidil* without a prescription at virtually all drugstores or supermarkets. It works well for small balding patches that you catch early. It takes a couple of months to show improvement, and you have to keep using it to keep the new hair coming. It is easy to apply and isn't greasy, so if you have a balding patch that you'd like to see improved, you might want to consider it.

Finasteride, a prescription ingredient known by the product name Propecia, is available as a pill—but is only for men with certain types of male pattern hair loss.

As for washing and conditioning your hair, good inexpensive drugstore shampoos are as wonderful as the expensive brands often found in salons—and in many cases, the drugstore ones work better.

The products that have really made a difference for hair in the last couple of decades have been those that contain some form of silicone for lubricating and smoothing frizzy hair, and adding lots of shine. These silicone-containing products usually have an ingredient listed within in the first few ingredients that end with the letters "*cone*," such as *cyclomethicone* or *dimethicone*. The first one we recall discovering years ago was the drugstore brand, "Frizz Ease," now called John Frieda Frizz Ease Hair Serum. You spread a couple of drops around your palms, then run your hands through your clean, damp hair. It's a great tangle remover and good for little girls' tangled hair, too—no more tears when combing after the bath!

Some shampoos and conditioners have silicone-based products already in them, and there are many brands and various concentrations, so you will want to experiment a bit as some of the serums are heavier than others. Using a "shine spray" with silicone may work better, as they won't weigh as much on the hair. Quite a few of the drugstore brands have both frizz serums and/or sprays, and finding the right preparation and amount for your exact needs will take a little experimentation.

It helps to protect your hair with one of those silicone products before you expose it to blow-dryers or straightening rods, but you can't depend on any product to completely protect your hair. Over-processed (colored or straightened, etc.) can create damaged, dry, dull, broken hair. Try to find a hairstyle that requires as little torture to your hair as possible.

Some people absolutely insist on having blonde hair, even though that means stripping the hair of its natural color first, then putting another one or two processes of color on top of that. Then they use heat styling tools. The blonde hair often comes out looking like a brittle bunch of straw—no shine or luster at all. Is that really what they had in mind?

Choice of hairstyle and color is such a personal decision— if someone is happy with a certain look and it makes them feel better to wear their hair a certain way, then we're all for it. We're pointing out the damage process because many people don't understand that it is *what they are doing to their hair* that causes the lack of luster and shine—the same way people often don't understand why their skin lacks clarity or luster. The fact is, they have not yet invented a product that can give you "natural blonde" luster the products are most likely the culprit that is taking away your healthy-looking hair.

They can put a man on the moon, but they can't find come up with perfect beauty products. You think it would be the most important thing on scientists' minds next to solving world hunger, right?

Arms and Legs, Elbows, Knees.

We already covered the truth about cellulite in the previous section, but the good news is that there is a lot you can do to give yourself lovely skin all over your body. If you have dry, rough knees and elbows, or bumpy, pimply skin on the back of your arms or other places on your body, you will notice a change in a few days if you follow some simple instructions.

The first important thing you need to know is YOU DON'T NEED DIFFERENT LOTIONS FOR OTHER BODY PARTS. Your face moisturizer is fabulous everywhere and anywhere. All that great real estate being used up in your bathroom for various hand, foot, eye and face lotions? Unnecessary! Reclaim your territory!

We understand the attraction of having different creams or perfumed lotions—all we're saying is that you don't *have* to have different ones. And same with your soap--Dove, baby. Dove all over. If you use the Dove Sensitive Skin preparation, you'll likely find that you won't get itchy under your arms or in other more sensitive areas, either. You'd be surprised how many people find a sudden "cure" for itchy issues just by switching soaps!

> As we mentioned before—always use a clean, dry washcloth. And if you use scrubbing gloves or a brush, be sure they are made of bacteria-resistant material and you let them dry completely between each use.

One of the best ways to get smooth skin is to give your-self a good cleaning with nylon bath or shower gloves (also called loofah gloves). The Body Shop has some that are pretty great. We've also seen these kinds of gloves in some drugstores. They last a long time and don't build up mildew.

Simply lather up the gloves with Dove and give yourself a really good rubdown, concentrating on the back of your arms and legs where those bumps are. Washcloths don't pro-vide the exfoliation power you need on those places, so use those gloves or a good stiff brush or loofah. Hit your bumpy and pimply areas with the gloves every day for a week and watch how quickly they disappear.

You might like to follow a good salt or sugar scrub—but again—think of exfoliation, not irritation.

Be sure you moisturize all over your body as soon as you towel off—this helps preserve more moisture in the skin.

After a good all-over scrub, your skin will immediately feel better and breathe better. You have sloughed off a whole lot of dead skin cells and the pores are open and breathing the air and fresh moisture you are providing.

More about the bumps on the back of arms and thighs, and your rough elbows and knees...

Let's address those bumps and rough patches a bit more. If you have a lot of them and they don't disappear after a week of exfoliation and moisturizing, you can perform a mini-Peel on them. For a mini-Peel on the backs of arms and legs, you might like to use a stronger percentage of glycolic acid, perhaps as high as a 50% solution. After all, the skin on your arms and legs is far tougher than the skin on your face, and needs a little stronger treatment. Use common sense and let your own body be the guide.

Simply apply your glycolic acid to the bumpy patches and rough elbows or knees after your scrub-down. Leave it on for about five minutes then rinse and dry off and follow with moisturizing. Every other day, repeat the scrub-down and evaluate the patches. If they are peeling or irritated, apply your moisturizer and wait a couple of days before scrubbing and evaluating again. Your skin's reaction will guide you on when to attempt the mini-Peel again.

After two to four weeks of scrubbing and mini-Peels, you should see significant improvement in those problem areas.

> You should not use *tretinoin* or *hydroquinone* all over your body, but you can safely use *glycolic acid* preparations on targeted areas of your body.

There are lots of body lotions that have 4% or 8% *glycolic* acid preparations in them, and you can get good ones we suggest on the web, or some in the drugstore. You might like to use those for all-over body maintenance after you have cured your bumpy or pimply or rough patches. You can always perform the stronger mini-Peel glycolic treatments if any problems start to recur.

And recall what we said about the bitter taste of *glycolic acid* preparations: Don't use them if you are going to get romantic!

The chest

The skin on your chest may or may not be thicker than the skin on your face, but it certainly isn't as hardy as the skin on your arms and legs. Use the scrub gloves lightly on your chest and underarms, and use extra moisturizer. If you have pimples on your chest—which is common if you have facial acne—you might find performing a *glycolic-acid* mini-Peel as described for arms and legs every week or so will keep the acne under control. If the acne is widespread and unsightly on your chest, then consult a dermatologist who can recommend products specifically for acne care.

Hands, Feet, and Nails

Oh, the hands! The old adage, "You can tell a woman's real age by looking at her hands," is still true. There is, to date, nothing to keep the thinner skin on the hands from becoming less elastic and wrinkled. But there is a lot you can do for age-spots and dryness.

The *hydroquinone* you use in The Skin Regime will work well on discoloration or age-spots on the hands. If you have very dry skin on the hands, you might like to get a lotion that contains a preparation with 8% to 16% *glycolic acid*—many drugstore brands have glycolic acid products.

As for nails—treat them with care, keep them moisturized.

Let's talk a moment about those cuticles on the nails. The cuticles serve as a barrier against infection. When you cut or otherwise damage them, it allows water to get in and possibly breed bacteria. We know they get dry and unruly, but try not to disrupt their natural state too much. Massage moisturizer into the nail beds, and maybe drop some mineral oil on them for extra lubrication. If you absolutely can't resist trimming the cuticles a little, then please use very clean utensils and proceed carefully.

If you use polish, try to limit how often you change colors, as polish removers really dry out the cuticles and nail beds. If you don't like to use polish, consider lightly buffing the nail for shine—buffer sticks or blocks are available at nearly any drugstore.

If you have weak nails that never grow without breaking, you might consider some of the new salon techniques for enhanced or false nails. Remember the days of acrylic nails? They still exist, but they have never been successful for everyone—they lift off, break, and often cause fungus problems. The latest trend is the use of UV Gels, which is applied in a similar technique used with acrylics, but UV Gels have a far better success rate of staying on and being trouble-free.

> Slather on sunblock on your hands before getting UV gels on the nails. It will help prevent age spots and other issues associated with UV lights.

UV Gels are applied with brushes. Then your nails are placed under an ultra-violet light for a few minutes. After the new nails are applied, they can be painted or buffed to look completely natural. Some salons have given up on acrylics and switched completely over to UV Gels.

Note: If you have never tried UV Gels and are planning to, you should know the light heats up the nail and you may feel a "burning sensation." If this happens, pull the nails out from under the light until it cools; the sensation will disappear quickly.

Now we are going to get the bottom of it all: The feet.

Don't spend lots of money on creams for cracked heels or anything claiming to be "just for" the feet—they are not necessary because they have nearly identical ingredients as other moisturizers. Sometimes a cooling-agent such as menthol or eucalyptus is used in foot preparations, and if you enjoy that then go ahead and use them. But for simply treating rough or dry skin, using The Hand and Foot Skin Regime for the hands and feet—as we describe below—will do the trick. You can use the same products you use for your face.

Here is the Hand and Foot Skin Regime for keeping your extremities soft and good-looking.

The Hand and Foot Skin Regime:

1. First exfoliate: For the hands, use a nail brush or loofah or your scrub gloves to smooth your skin and get rid of dead skin cells. For your feet, first use a good callous filer, paying closer attention to the heels and balls of your feet. You can get a good coarse filer at a beauty supply store or at the drugstore, such as those made by Dr. Scholl's. Filing is the best way to smooth out the cracked heels and rough skin.

2. Follow with a good sugar or salt scrub if you wish.

3. Apply a layer of 8 - 15% *glycolic acid* lotion on the hands and feet.

4. Let the *glycolic acid* lotion settle in for a few minutes, then apply a very generous layer of your moisturizer, being sure to massage into your cuticles.

5. Finally, slather on a layer of mineral oil or Vaseline, massage into cuticles of finger and toenails, and place plastic bags (such as Baggies, or any other inexpensive food-storage bag) over your hands and feet—but don't try to walk with the Baggies on, you'll slip!

6. Relax and let the moisture layers soak in for 10-20 minutes, then wipe off excess oil or Vaseline.

If you have a lot of cracking on your heels or thick calluses on the feet, repeat the Hand and Foot Regime every couple of days and you'll find an amazing difference in a very short time.

If you have truly neglected your feet and have corns and calluses so thick that they don't respond to your filing, consider a visit to the podiatrist to get you on the road, then maintain with the Hand and Foot Regime after.

A Word About Perfume.

Perfume is a lovely touch—a gorgeous scent to compliment your gorgeous skin.

Keep in mind that perfume is a type of makeup—an invisible makeup. Ages ago, scented oils and perfumes were intended to help hide the stench of body odors for humans that were unable to bathe frequently. Perfumes were used by men and women alike.

Of course, this meant you had really stinky people with heavy layers of perfume. And sometimes on the subway in the summer in the city, it appears there are a lot of people still following that ages-old method of perfume use.

> With perfume, as with makeup: Subtle is sexier.

But we shall assume you follow modern hygiene procedures and you think of perfume as an accessory or adornment. Therefore, you should use perfume to <u>enhance</u>, not to hide. A delicate wisp of pleasant scent is attractive and non-offensive, but pouring it on heavily never pleases anyone. You end up repelling people instead of attracting them—as if you put on a bug-spray for humans! And you can't always trust your own nose to know when you are overdoing it, as you quickly get used to the scent you have put on and may not realize you are putting on too much.

So keep this in mind: An oil-based scent will last longer than quickly-evaporating alcohol-based products. A little dab in heat-releasing areas such as behind the ears or under the breasts is all you need. If you fear the scent will evaporate during the day, choose to carry a little atomizer with you rather than putting it on too heavy in the morning in the hopes it will last all day.

If it is a spray scent, try spritzing a little in the air in front of you and then stepping into the mist. This way, your clothing and hair will absorb just the right amount. Avoid spraying directly on to your skin or clothing—that will almost always be too much.

A word about the neglected areas.

Clean them once in a while, even though they are so easy to overlook. Let all your skin breath and get healthy! Give a swipe with your scrub gloves between your toes, behind and around the curves of your ears, your butt crack and your ankles. And your bellybutton—you know what starts fermenting in there? Get a cotton swab and clean it out once in a while. We know no one sees your skin in these places (or *do* they?) but you have to live in your skin and so you might as well take good care of it—for yourself, if not for someone else.

Handy Shopping List

Take this list with you to the drugstore or health food store, or keep handy as you look search on the internet.

Also visit TheSkinRegime.com for resources.

MUST HAVE ITEMS:

--Rough washcloths (or cheap dishtowels cut into squares)

--Dove Sensitive Skin Beauty Bar. Alternate item: Cetaphil Daily Facial Cleanser

--Lubriderm Sensitive Skin Therapy Lotion. Alternate item: Cetaphil Moisturizing Cream

--SUNSCREEN for anyone who spends more than a few minutes a day with exposure to the sun

--Glycoloic Acid Peels, 20% or higher peel solutions. Go to TheSkinRegime.com for resources.

--Rubbing Alcohol (or pre-peel preparations if your Peel comes with it).

OPTIONAL ITEMS:

--(optional for Maintenance) prescription for tretinoin cream (Retin-A).

--(optional, for people who have some acne) Benzoyl peroxide 10% cream, such as made by Clearasil

--(optional, for people with melasma/dark spots) prescription for hydroquinone 4% cream.

--(optional, for people who may develop some irritation) Antibacterial cream with pain reliever "pramoxine HCl, such as found in some Bacitraycin or Neosporin products. Often found in the first-aid aisle.

--(optional) Fish oil and Vitamins

--(optional) large cotton balls or cotton squares for applying glycolic acid preparations

--(optional) latex or non-latex disposable gloves. Often in first-aid aisles, or ask pharmacist

ABOUT THE AUTHOR:

Dana Ramos is a skin-care enthusiast and writer who lives in Westchester, New York. She's from California where she obtained a Masters in Professional Writing from USC and wrote screenplays (a requirement for California residency). In addition to creating and writing **The Skin Regime** book and concept, she writes freelance articles and is working on other books (a requirement for New York residency). Visit DanaRamos.com for more information. And TheSkinRegime.com

    Dr. David Bank is the founder and head of The Center for Dermatology, Cosmetic and Laser Surgery in Mount Kisco, New York. His patient list contains famous names as well as regular people (like Dana!). He is frequently called on as a source for television shows such as The Today Show, Good Morning America, and magazines--including Vogue, Elle and Allure. He is a former President of the New York State Society for Dermatology and Dermatologic Surgery. Visit TheCenterforDerm.com for more information about Dr. Bank and The Center.

THANK YOU TO:

Ester Hacken for advice and encouragement, proofreading and spurring me on. She also has a super website of toys and goodies at Blumonga.com

My wonderful children for being the jewels they are, and my late husband, Douglas, for 27 years of love and support for everything I pursued in life.

To the terrific friends and family who lent their time—and faces—to test products and give opinions, and finally proving enthusiastically that The Skin Regime works—it really really works!

Dr. David Bank for providing valuable information and insights for this book, kind honesty and integrity, and wonderful dermatological care for many years.

Extra info:

TheSkinRegime.com
   The latest news on the TRUTH about skin care products, as well as products and guides to finding the best product for you. Sign up for our newsletter!

American Academy of Dermatology: AAD.org
   Lots of the techno-geek info if you want to read the science behind everything in skin care.

Skin Cancer Foundation: SkinCancer.org
   The leading skin cancer prevention and information organization.

MakeupAlley.com
   A fun place to read about newest products and reader reviews on makeup.

And visit TheSkinRegime.com for more updated info on resources and extra information.

Made in the USA
Lexington, KY
09 October 2012